# THE STRU
# OF THE
# NATIONAL HEALTH
# SERVICE

*by*
## *Tracey Jones*

**Practice Premises/Staff Adviser to Avon Health
Authority**

**PUBLISHING
INITIATIVES
BOOKS**

**Doral House • 2(b) Manor Road
Beckenham • Kent • BR3 5LE**

# ACKNOWLEDGEMENTS

I gratefully acknowledge the support and assistance of the following people in the production of this book:-

| | |
|---|---|
| *Paul Frisby* | Planning Manager, Frenchay NHS Trust |
| *Linda Ewles* | Health Promotion Commissioning Manager Avon Health Authority |
| *Pat Turton* | Department of Social Medicine, University of Bristol |
| *Dammy Le Grand* | Bristol Social Services |
| *Catherine Beale* | South & West NHSE Regional Office |

Special thanks also goes to:-

| | |
|---|---|
| *Sarah Allen* | Avon Health Authority |
| *Yvonne Monks* | Avon Health Authority |
| *David Perkins* | United Bristol Healthcare NHS Trust |

**First published** January 1995
**Second edition** March 1997

*Printed by:*

Hamlet Press
7-9 Westfield Street
London SE18

**ISBN**
1 873839 17 0

Further copies of *The Structure of The National Health Service* may be obtained from Pi books, a division of Publishing Initiatives (Europe) Ltd. This publication reflects the view and experience of the author, and not necessarily those of the Publisher.

# FOREWORD

There exists a belief among some health-care educationalists that everyone working within the NHS has a comprehensive working knowledge of its structure and constituent parts. I believe the opposite may be true for, unlike other large organisations where employees do have sound ideas of roles and functions, this becomes more difficult within the NHS because of the continual changes imposed upon it. Therefore, gaining an understanding of our multi-faceted NHS will be of tremendous value to all levels of staff, enabling them to see the whole picture and, importantly, their place within it. This is as true for someone who has worked in this environment for years as for someone new to the field.

Within this world, where change seems to be the only constant, the author ably leads us to an understanding of the vocabulary of purchasers, providers, budgets, the internal market etc., with clear usage of both past and current models of the various component parts, starting with the NHSE - familiar to many staff only as a set of initials on the directives they receive. This chapter leaves the reader with a clear overview of the top of the hierarchical structure, which we can begin to relate to ourselves and our role.

The excellent in-depth analysis of the differing roles of the HA clearly demonstrates its influence on a day-to-day basis and provides a comprehensive guide to an organisation still viewed by many as merely the paymaster responding to claims submitted, or the supplier of stationery. We are led logically to the NHS Trusts and services with a clear definition of the role of these health-care providers. Social services has also recently undergone much change, particularly so since the introduction of the *Community Care Act* 1990, becoming an integral part of primary care and destined to play an even greater role in future services development. Encouragingly, the author includes the *Health and Safety at Work Act* which is a cornerstone of good practice, emphasising each individual's responsibilities in his/her work environment.

It is generally assumed that only staff working in a fundholding practice understand its function and aims; however, I believe that all levels of staff will gain some benefit from this clear description of the scheme. Importantly, the emerging growth area of complementary therapists has also been included as nowadays they work in close harmony with more traditional medicine.

This volume has many good qualities: it flows logically, is well written and is comprehensive. Yet perhaps above all else its best quality is the way it makes the hitherto little-understood structure of the NHS available to us all and will encourage all staff to appreciate the potentially major role their discipline has to play in future health-care provision.

*Pauline Webdale MAMS, Dip PM*
Practice Manager, Chairman of the National Council of AMSPAR

# CONTENTS

# GLOSSARY

| | |
|---|---|
| *Antenatal* | Before birth. |
| *Auditor General* | One who audits accounts. |
| *Basic Practice Allowance* | A payment to GPs who have more than 1,200 patients on their list. |
| *Cash-Limited (Budget)* | Not open-ended, a set amount of money which cannot be increased. |
| *Cochlear Implant* | Electrode implanted into the cavity of the internal ear. |
| *Comptroller* | One who checks expenditure. |
| *Dietetic* | Of diet. |
| *Doctors' Deputising Service* | Service used by GPs to cover out-of-hours visits, i.e. nights and weekends. |
| *Epidemiology* | Study of diseases usually prevalent among a community at a particular time (epidemics). |
| *Executive Members* | Members of a Committee or Board who are full-time officers/directors of the organisation. |
| *Hardship Dispensing Lists* | Patients whose drugs are dispensed to them by their GP, providing they live more than a mile away from a chemist, because they suffer from some form of disability/impairment. |
| *Items of Service* | Services provided to the patients by GPs, e.g. maternity, emergency treatment, vaccinations and immunisations. |
| *Lipid Disorders* | High levels of fat or cholesterol in the blood stream. Often genetic. |
| *Medical Audit* | Audit within practices. |
| *Minor Surgery* | The following surgical procedures, e.g. injections - varicose veins, aspirations - cysts, incisions - warts, removal of foreign bodies. |
| *Morbidity* | Prevalence of disease. |
| *Non-Cash-Limited (Budget)* | An open-ended budget, not a set amount. |
| *Non-Executive Members* | Members of a Committee or Board who are not officers/directors of the organisation. |
| *Obstetricians* | Doctors specialising in childbirth. |

| | |
|---|---|
| *Orthodontics* | Correction of irregularities in teeth. |
| *Palliative* | Way of alleviating a disease without curing. |
| *Patients' Charter* | Includes such rights as the right to be registered with a GP, change GP quickly and easily, receive a copy of your GP's practice leaflet etc. |
| *Postnatal* | After birth. |
| *Postgraduate Education Allowance* | A payment to GPs who have attended 25 days of accredited postgraduate education. During this time they must have attended at least two accredited courses in: Health Promotion and the Prevention of Illness; Disease Management; Service Management. |
| *Practice Annual Report* | These provide data on consultation rates, hospital referrals, morbidity etc. |
| *Practice-Based Formularies* | An agreement within a practice that GPs will only prescribe from an agreed list of drugs. |
| *Prescription Exemption* | Exemption from payment for prescription due to age, income or medical condition. |
| *Psychophysical* | The relationship between mind and body. |
| *Rent and Rate Reimbursement* | The reimbursement of either an actual or notional rent to GPs for occupying their practice premises. Rates and water rates are also reimbursed. |
| *Ring Fencing* | An amount of money which has to be used for that purpose and that purpose alone |
| *Sickle Cell Anaemia* | A form of anaemia where the red blood cells are sickle-shaped. An abnormal form of haemoglobin is present. |
| *Stomacare* | A method of passing urine or faeces out of the body, through the intestine wall, rather than through the usual orifices. |
| *Temporary Residents* | A patient who needs to see a GP while away from home, e.g. while staying with friend, on business, etc. |
| *Tinnitus* | Ringing in the ears. |
| *Toxaemia* | Forms of blood poisoning. |
| *Trainee Payment* | A payment made to GPs for training another practitioner. |
| *Urology* | The treatment of disorders and diseases of the kidneys, ureters, bladder, prostate and urethra. |

# ABBREVIATIONS

| | |
|---|---|
| A&E | Accident and Emergency |
| AIDS | Acquired Immune Deficiency Syndrome |
| BMAS | British Medical Acupuncture Society |
| CESDI | Confidential Enquiry into Stillbirths and Deaths in Infants |
| CHC | Community Health Council |
| CPN | Community Psychiatric Nurse |
| CRDC | Central Research and Development Committee |
| CRMF | Cancer Relief MacMillan Fund |
| CT | Computerised Tomography |
| DHA | District Health Authority |
| DMU | Directly Managed Unit |
| DoH | Department of Health |
| DPO | Dental, Pharmaceutical and Ophthalmic |
| ECG | Electrocardiogram |
| ECR | Extra-Contractual Referral |
| FHS | Family Health Services |
| FHSA | Family Health Services Authority |
| GMS | General Medical Services |
| GP | General Practitioner |
| HA | Health Authority |
| HCHS | Hospital and Community Health Services |
| HIS | Health Information Service |
| HIV | Human Immunodeficiency Virus |
| HSE | Health and Safety Executive |
| HSWA | *Health and Safety at Work Act* |
| IT | Information Technology |

| | |
|---|---|
| *JCC* | Joint Consultative Committee |
| *MIND* | National Association for Mental Health |
| *MRI* | Magnetic Resonance Imaging |
| *NAHAT* | National Association of Health Authorities and Trusts |
| *NBA* | National Blood Authority |
| *NHS* | National Health Service |
| *NHSE* | National Health Service Executive |
| *NVQ* | National Vocational Qualification |
| *OHD* | Occupational Health Department |
| *OT* | Occupational Therapy |
| *PES* | Public Expenditure Survey |
| *PGEA* | Postgraduate Education Allowance |
| *PHCT* | Primary Health-Care Team |
| *RCN* | Royal College of Nursing |
| *R&D* | Research and Development |
| *RGN* | Registered General Nurse |
| *RHA* | Regional Health Authority |
| *RN* | Registered Nurse |
| *RNIB* | Royal National Institute for the Blind |
| *RNID* | Royal National Institute for the Deaf |
| *RTC* | Regional Transfusion Centre |
| *SHA* | Special Health Authority |
| *SHO* | Senior House Officer |
| *SRN* | State Registered Nurse |
| *STAT* | Society of Teachers of the Alexander Technique |
| *STG* | Special Transitional Grant |
| *UKCC* | United Kingdom Central Council for Nursing, Midwifery and Health Visiting |

# INTRODUCTION

This book is designed to give an outline to the structure of the National Health Service (NHS) and the changes it is undergoing. It also gives a comprehensive breakdown of all the constituent parts in a format designed to give information on the following areas:

- What the body/organisation is.
- How it is organised.
- What are its chief aims.
- What it does.
- What services it provides.

There then follows a number of shorter chapters on a variety of subjects which, while still relevant to general practice, are not perhaps part of the more basic structure of the NHS.

Whilst the NHS is still undergoing a period of change and settling into its new-found joint purchaser role, all Family Health Services Authorities (FHSAs) and District Health Authorities (DHAs) have now merged to form Health Authorities (HAs).

All Regional Health Authorities (RHAs) have now been absorbed within the National Health Service Executive Regional Offices.

It is difficult to talk about various organisations without going into a certain amount of detail and using as a model those organisations with which I have the greatest communication. It is, therefore, important to point out that the individual chapters should be treated as what is generally the norm within these organisations, and that there will always be certain exceptions to the rule. Section headings and departmental titles should also only be used as a guide to how a particular body might be organised, as there is a regional variation in structure. It is, therefore, appropriate to take note of the aims of the organisations and the functions they perform, rather than the names of individual directorates or departments.

In addition, when talking about NHS Trusts, I have tended to focus on those Trusts that provide acute and general medical services (former district hospitals). However, in many localities the ambulance service operates as a Trust, and many Trusts have responsibility for providing health-care facilities for people with learning difficulties.

The changes the NHS has gone through during the past two years have had success in bringing about more direct access to public health advice by GPs, greater collaboration between hospital and community services for fundholders and non-fundholders alike, and an integrated and improved primary and secondary care interface.

Since the introduction of the *Patients' Charter* and the increase in public awareness of what the NHS can, and possibly should, provide, greater pressure has been placed upon practice receptionists to have an increased understanding of the structure of the NHS. In order to assist with the quality of service offered to patients, it is essential that practice receptionists are aware of certain changes to the NHS, such as the difference between fundholding and non-fundholding practices, or the lines of accountability and funding within the NHS. The practice receptionist is usually the patient's first, and often most frequent, point of contact with the NHS. It is imperative to understand that, while maintaining individuality, the receptionist is part of a team working to provide the best possible primary and secondary care available. It is often all too easy for receptionists to act unilaterally, and to forget that they are part of a much larger organisation with far-reaching goals.

Finally, I must stress that any views contained within the book are my own and not necessarily the view of Avon Health Authority.

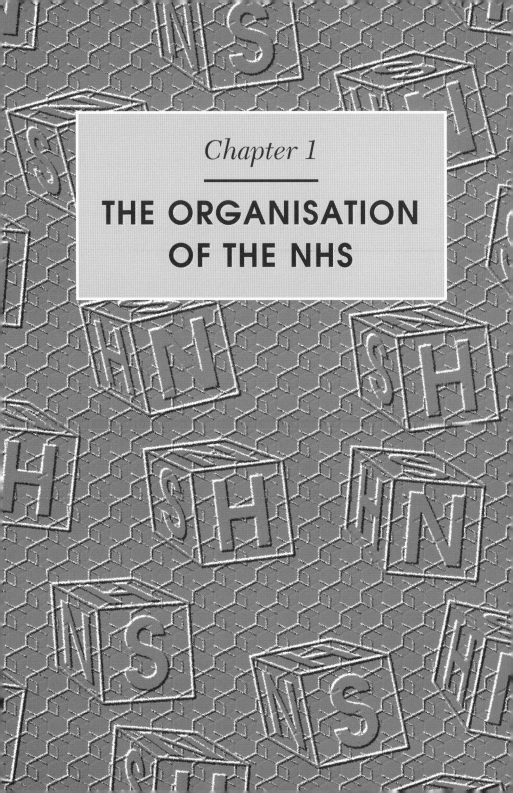

*Chapter 1*

# THE ORGANISATION OF THE NHS

Up until recently, the organisational structure of the NHS was as follows (see Figure 1). Whilst it is still undergoing a period of change, the current organisational structure is as shown in Figure 2 (p. 16).

At the top of the structure is the Secretary of State for Health, who is in fact the Minister responsible for the Department of Health (DoH). Also within this department is a Minister of State and a number of Junior Ministers.

The broad strategic direction of the NHS is set by a policy board, which is chaired by the Secretary of State.

The NHS Executive (NHSE) deals with all operational matters within the strategy and directives set by the policy board. The NHSE comprises a Chief Executive, Permanent Secretary and Chief Medical Officer. There are then approximately 4,500 civil servants. The key functions of the Department of Health are:

a) To establish the policy framework for the NHS. Major policy statements are usually delivered through Government White Papers. The DoH also publishes guidance on priorities and planning, and it is these documents that Authorities and Trusts refer to when preparing their own future plans.

b) To negotiate the level of NHS funding with the Treasury. The DoH retains some resources to run its own department and fund statutory bodies, such as the National Blood Authority and NHS Supplies Authority. However, the vast majority of its budget is now in effect distributed to Health Authorities.

c) To monitor the performance of NHS Authorities and Trusts, through the Regional Offices, and to assess the way in which they use their resources. For Health Authorities this means an ongoing discussion between members of the NHSE and their regional counterparts, culminating in a corporate contract which is agreed between the Chief Executive of the NHSE and each Regional Office and Chief Executive of the Health Authority.

The performance of NHS Trusts is also monitored by the eight outposts of the NHS Executive. This involves the assessment of the Trust's performance against the business plan it has produced.

## NEW NHS STRUCTURE

In October 1993, the Government announced plans to change the structure of the NHS in England.

The three key elements of the change were:

a) the merger of DHAs and FHSAs
b) the abolition of RHAs
c) a streamlined NHSE operating through eight Regional Offices.

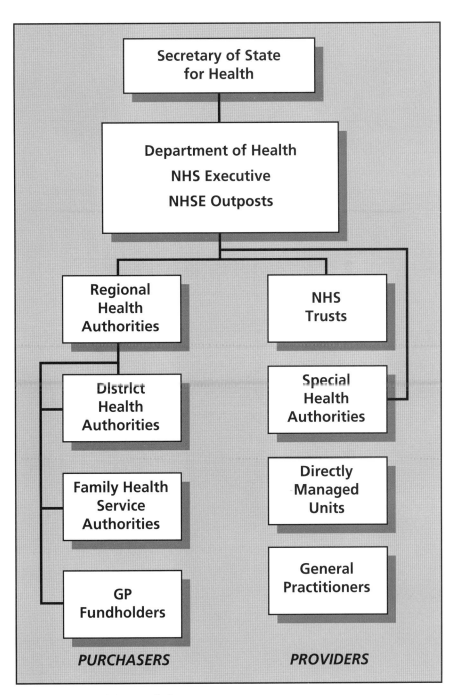

Fig 1. Structure of the NHS before 1994

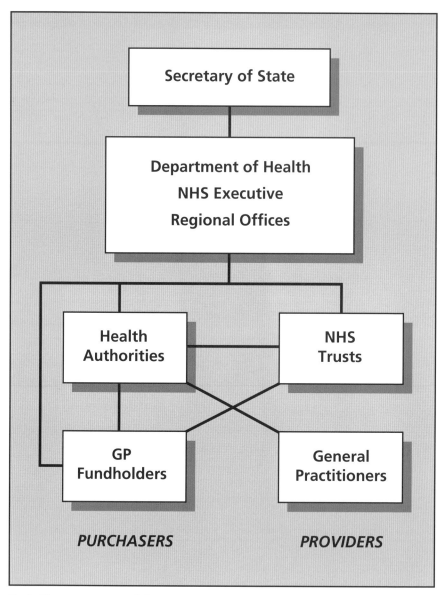

Fig 2. *The new structure of the NHS*

The main rationale behind the restructuring was to reduce management costs and to direct a greater proportion of the NHS budget towards direct patient care.

These changes actually came into effect on the 1st April 1996. The eight Regional Health Authorities which previously existed have now been fully absorbed within the NHSE Regional Offices (see Figures 3 and 4).

The NHSE Regional Offices have increased their responsibilities to include most of the functions that have in the past been carried out by RHAs. In effect, this means that the NHSE becomes responsible for relating to both 'purchasers' and 'providers'.

NHSE Regional Offices no longer comprise a board of executive and non-executive directors, but are part of the Executive. NHSE Regional Directors report directly to the NHS Chief Executive, and form the Executive Board. As the NHSE is now part of the civil service there are no non-executive members present except the Chairman. This role involves:

- Holding meetings with chairpeople of Health Authorities and Trusts covered by the relevant Regional Office, and acting as a channel of communication to and from the Secretary of State.

- Acting as an adviser to the Secretary of State on the appointment and reappointment of chairpeople and non-executive directors in the region.

- Acting as a mentor to chairpeople in the region, especially when newly appointed, in the business of chairing and leading a public body.

The merger of DHAs and FHSAs has created an integrated purchasing authority at local level.

The main aim of streamlining the Executive is to enable it and the DoH to concentrate on head office functions and supporting Ministers, and enable purchasers and providers to take the lead in the management of local services.

## WHITLEY COUNCIL

When the NHS was formed in 1948, it was agreed that a system of Whitley Councils (named after J.H. Whitley, who chaired a 1917 committee into ways of securing permanent improvements in industrial relations) should be created to enable employees' views to be taken into account before decisions were made on levels of pay and conditions of service.

The first Whitley Councils were established in 1950, and by 1974 they had evolved into 10 functional councils responsible for one or more major NHS staff groups, and a general council responsible for the conditions of service which are common to all staff.

Doctors' and dentists' remuneration is, however, decided at Cabinet level after advice has been taken from the independent Doctors' and Dentists' Review Body. A number of other professional groups, such as nursing staff, midwives, health visitors and professionals allied to medicine, also operate in this manner.

In addition, although there is an agreed scale, many individual Chief Executives' pay is determined by individual Health Authorities within this range. The result of this is that approximately 40% of NHS staff have their pay determined by the

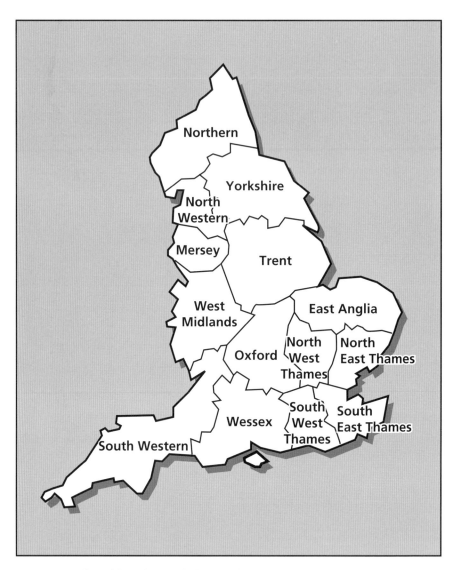

*Fig 3. Regional Health Authorities before April 1994*

Whitley system, while the other 60% depend upon pay review bodies and local Health Authorities.

The main exceptions to this rule are NHS Trusts, who, apart from the salaries of junior hospital doctors, have freedom to depart from the nationally established rates of pay.

Within GP practices there has generally been a move away from Whitley Council grades and terms and conditions of service for newly appointed staff.

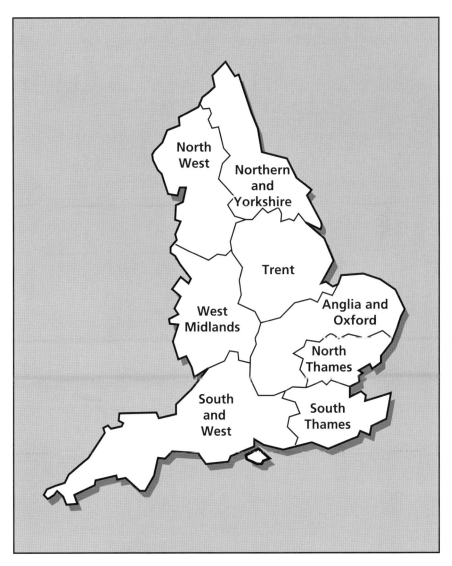

*Fig 4. New NHSE Regional Offices since 1st April 1996.*

## THE STRUCTURE OF THE NHS IN WALES AND SCOTLAND

The NHS in Wales comprises five integrated Health Authorities. These Health Authorities work directly with the Welsh Office as there is no regional tier in between.

The main policy document for Wales is entitled *A fresh start*. This document, in line with its counterparts in England, is an attempt to secure a primary care led NHS.

Another document worth mentioning is *Caring for the future* which provides the basis for the performance management agreements between the DoH, Welsh Health Authorities and Trusts.

In Scotland the current Chief Executive of the NHS Management Executive is also the Chief Executive of the Department of Health. A public health policy unit which is separate from the Management Executive, but part of the DoH, is headed up by the Chief Medical Officer.

The Scottish DoH comprises 15 Health Boards and 47 Trusts which report to the Secretary of State for Scotland through the Management Executive.

What is different about the Scottish health-care system is that due to its sparsely populated islands it has maintained a number of Directly Managed Units (DMUs). In addition, it has been slow to adopt fundholding in a major way.

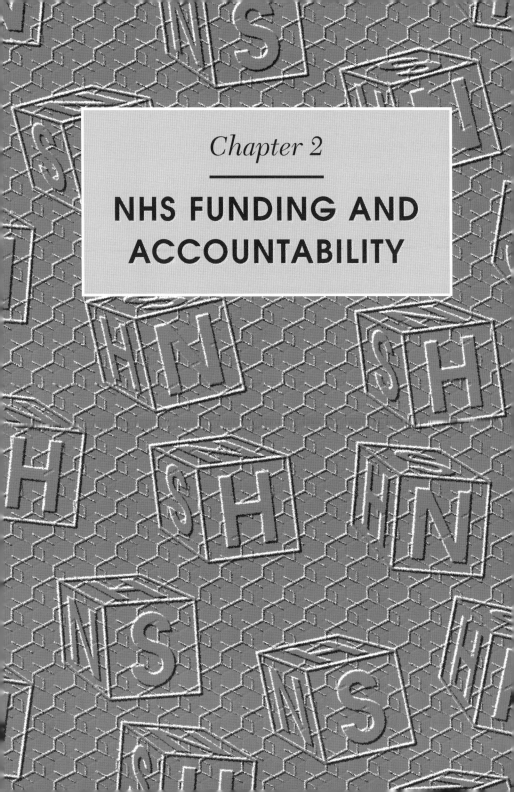

# Chapter 2

---

# NHS FUNDING AND ACCOUNTABILITY

Currently, the NHS accounts for 15% of government expenditure (see Figure 5). The system by which each government department's spending needs are assessed is known as the Public Expenditure Survey (PES).

The cycle starts with ministers bidding for funding for the next three years for their particular department. These bids, once they have been formulated, are then discussed with the Treasury. The agreed levels of public sector spending are then announced by the Chancellor of the Exchequer in his Autumn Statement.

In the past, most NHS funding has come from Parliament out of general taxation. Although this trend has continued, greater emphasis is now placed on NHS contributions, patient charges and miscellaneous income. The agreed overall budget is then split between hospital and community services, and family health services.

Particular policies or programmes take priority. Examples include waiting list initiatives, acquired immune deficiency syndrome (AIDS) programmes and out-of-hours development.

## BUDGET ALLOCATION

The national formula for working out the amount of funding received by Health Authorities has changed since the April 1996 reforms. This has meant that many authorities, such as Avon, which have previously received a reasonable amount of growth money, have received no growth and only an inflation increase for this and, probably, coming financial years.

The funding which comes from the DoH is classified as 'hospital and community health services' (HCHS) and family health services (FHS). The budget allocation received by Health Authorities will, therefore, include both HCHS and FHS monies. FHS funding is a ring-fenced allocation and has both cash and non-cash limited elements to it. HCHS monies may be used to promote and improve General Medical Services, but FHS funding cannot be used to support HCHS.

## CAPITAL CHARGES

Funding for schemes such as investment in new equipment and repairs to hospitals are allocated separately from Health Authorities' revenues. Depending upon the size of the scheme these projects need the approval of the NHSE Regional Office, DoH or Treasury.

As a way to ensure that the NHS uses its capital more efficiently, there is now a charge for capital assets. Directly Managed Units (DMUs) no longer exist and thus only Trusts make capital charge payments, or interest and depreciation payments, to Health Authorities. Trusts will in turn make an increased charge to the cost of the services they provide to the purchaser units.

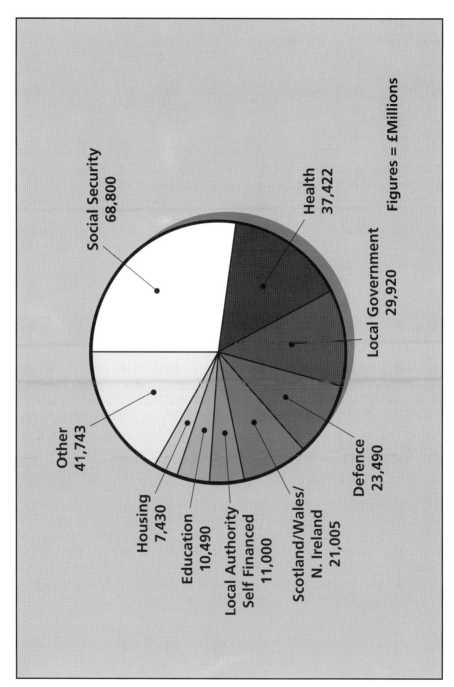

Social Security
68,800

Health
37,422

Local Government
29,920

Figures = £Millions

Other
41,743

Housing
7,430

Education
10,490

Local Authority
Self Financed
11,000

Scotland/Wales/
N. Ireland
21,005

Defence
23,490

*Fig 5. Public spending breakdown*

## ACCOUNTABILITY
### Parliamentary committees

Because the Secretary of State is responsible to Parliament for the NHS, MPs are able to raise questions and issues about it in the House of Commons. In short, this means that parliamentary accountability acts as a centralising influence. Examples of particular parliamentary committees are detailed below.

### *Public Accounts Committee*

The Public Accounts Committee investigates the way in which money voted by Parliament has been spent. It is supported in its role by the Comptroller and Auditor General, and the National Audit Office.

### *Health Committee of the House of Commons*

This committee shadows the work of the DoH and investigates major issues of health policy.

Both of these committees will take written and oral evidence from ministers, civil servants and NHS employees.

In addition, the Health Service Commissioner or Ombudsman is also an important figure. The main role of the Ombudsman is to investigate possible maladministration within the NHS. This may mean carrying out enquiries into the activities of NHS Authorities and Trusts. The results of these enquiries are made public.

### Audit Commission

This is an independent body set up by Act of Parliament to audit the NHS and local government. The Commission has produced a number of reports, which have resulted in the DoH implementing policies to improve the efficiency with which resources are used.

The fact that virtually all money for the NHS is voted by Parliament and is derived from taxes and National Insurance contributions, means that Parliament has an increasing interest in the running of the NHS.

However, as Authorities and Trusts comprise local people, they will often differ about the way it is felt ministerial policies should be put into practice. Authorities and Trusts do, therefore, maintain some scope for adapting national policies to suit local circumstances.

# Chapter 3

---

# NHSE REGIONAL OFFICES

Since the reforms of April 1996 the NHSE Regional Offices have taken on the roles of the old Regional Health Authorities. NHSE Regional Offices have a key strategic role in the management of the NHS. They are responsible for managing change, and for ensuring that government policies are implemented. Health Authorities are directly responsible to the NHSE Regional Offices.

The NHSE Regional Office comprises a Regional Chair and a number of Regional Directors. For example, in the South and West these are the Director of Performance Management, the Director of Finance and the Director of Public Health.

## KEY FUNCTIONS

The main functions of the NHS Regional Office are:

- Performance management of Health Authorities, including progress in implementing national policies and priorities through the NHS contracts with health-care providers and ensuring compliance with Minister's policies.
- Monitoring the performance of NHS Trusts against the agreed financial criteria, and in a limited number of non-financial areas which cannot be pursued through NHS Trusts.
- Advising on prioritisation for capital resources between Trust and non-Trust capital (including forward joint working with local authorities, the voluntary sector and primary-care infrastructure), and promoting the government's private finance initiatives.
- Approving capital investments in Trusts within the legislative limits.
- Approving applications to join the GP fundholding scheme and setting budgets for GP fundholders.
- Ensuring that the NHS internal market functions effectively.
- Liaising with universities in relation to medical and dental education.
- Setting the local research agenda within the national framework and managing the research and development programme.
- Workforce planning and commissioning of education and training.
- Establishing Community Health Councils.
- Developing the public health function at local level.
- Management and disposal of redundant properties.

The main role of the NHSE Regional Office is to manage the purchasing function. As previously stated, Health Authorities, which are seen as purchasing health-care services for their local populations, are directly accountable to NHSE Regional Offices. At present, GP fundholders are also accountable to NHSE Regional Offices in terms of their purchasing function. The budget offer comes from the Health Authority in the name of the Regional Office. The Regional Office also has a list of agreed items which can be purchased by fundholders. Really though, all the work and face-to-face contact is with the Health Authority.

In addition to distributing Health Authority resources, the NHSE Regional Office provides support and guidance to purchasers in the management of the internal market. It also monitors the management performance of Health Authorities to ensure that the most efficient and cost-effective balance of primary and secondary health-care services is obtained.

Within many regions, Health Authorities and Trusts are linked to region-wide information networks known as the 'clearing house system'. Inpatient, day-case, outpatient and waiting list data are gathered from providers' patient-administration systems each month and sent to the regional computer centre for processing. The information is validated by the regional information unit, and then made available to all purchasers within the region. The 'clearing house system' was designed to ensure that all purchasers and providers within a region have access to accurate information, which allows them to carry out medical audit, and public health and epidemiology projects.

## The *Patients' Charter*

The *Patients' Charter* promotes high standards of health care, through the implementation of rights and standards. It is a key objective of any NHSE Regional Office.

The main thrust of the document is to sustain and improve the standards that patients have a right to expect from the NHS. In addition, most authorities have published their own charters which include local recommended standards.

## Open Health

Some regions have launched an information service for members of the public and the NHS. **Open Health:**

**Health Information Service (HIS): Freephone - 0800 665544**
**Lines are open 9am - 5pm Monday-Friday**

The service provides information on a range of health matters, including:

• Local and national support groups
• NHS services
• Medical conditions
• Patients' rights

The main objectives of the service are to provide comprehensive health information to individuals in need - directly, through carers or through other health-care professionals. The service is provided free and is entirely confidential. The intention is that it complements the advice and recommendations of health professionals.

## NHSE HQ

The main functions are as follows:

- Supporting ministers in accounting for the performance of the NHS at a national level.

- Taking the lead in setting and maintaining the strategic framework and in policy development.

- Developing and evaluating the NHS research and development strategy.

- Securing resources and making allocations to Health Authorities.

- Developing and evaluating a strategy for outcomes which have been driven by evidence-based effective health care.

- Making capital allocations to providers and advising ministers on the balance between major schemes, non-Trust capital and block capital and ensuring, as part of the Government's Private Finance Initiative, that private finance alternatives are viewed as a standard option whenever capital schemes are considered.

- Developing national policies on human resources including education and training.

- Setting the overall framework for performance management including guidance on priorities.

- Developing and maintaining links with NHS in Wales, Scotland and Northern Ireland.

## SPECIAL HEALTH AUTHORITIES (SHAs)

Some NHS services are run by Special Health Authorities. Examples are the NHS Supplies Authority and the National Blood Authority. SHAs are directly responsible to the Secretary of State.

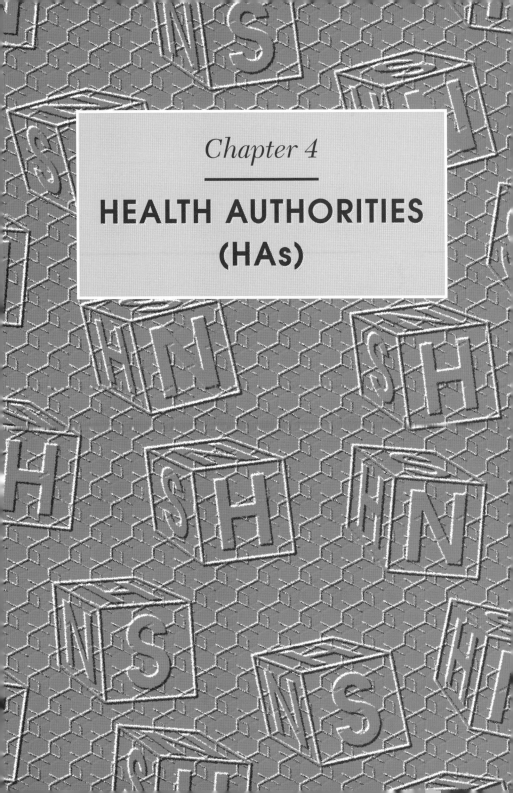

*Chapter 4*

# HEALTH AUTHORITIES
# (HAs)

Since April 1996 Health Authorities have used funds allocated to them by the NHSE to purchase primary and secondary care services. The management of these secondary care services is undertaken by NHS Trusts. These are often referred to as provider units. There are 100 Health Authorities in England with populations that range from 100,000 to over 800,000. The membership of the Health Authority comprises the Chairperson and a board of executives and non-executive directors. The Chief Executive of the Health Authority is an executive director.

---

## BOX 1 *THE MAIN FUNCTIONS OF THE HEALTH AUTHORITY*

Understanding the health status of the local population.

•

Co-ordinating health promotion efforts through a wide range of agencies.

•

Assessing the need for health services.

•

Purchasing health services to meet these needs as far as possible within the budget available.

•

Ensuring that the services provided are effective and of a high quality.

•

Planning the strategic development of health services with local NHS Trusts and GPs.

•

Administering the contracts of, and paying for the services provided by GPs, dentists, pharmacists and opticians.

•

Informing the public about the services these professionals provide.

•

Planning improvements and developments to services.

•

Investigating complaints made by members of the public about services provided by GPs.

---

## MAIN FUNCTIONS OF THE HEALTH AUTHORITY

The main functions of the HA are shown in Box 1. In order to fulfil this role the HA works closely with:

- Social services departments
- Unitary authorities
- GP fundholders

- Voluntary bodies
- NHS Trusts
- Community Health Councils.

Avon Health Authority is broken down into five directorates:

1. Contracting
2. Corporate Management
3. Development
4. Finance
5. Public Health.

The main responsibilities for each reorganised directorate are as follows:

## Contracting Directorate

- Negotiating and monitoring of contracts with the provider units.
- Joint commissioning in partnership with unitary authorities.
- Strategic implementation of agreed policies across all client groups.
- Contracting interface with GP fundholders.
- Nursing home registration.

Also linked to this Directorate is a Learning Difficulties Project Team.

## Corporate Management Directorate

- Developing the corporate work, communications, organisation and culture of the HA.
- Maintaining a close working relationship with the Chief Executive and Chairman using corporate contract, work programme, communications, and training and development mechanisms.
- Managing the administration of Board and Executive meetings.
- Overview of secretarial and support staff.
- The handling of public relations.
- Some personnel and house management functions.
- Dealing with statutory duties, such as complaints and corporate governance.

## Development Directorate

- Primary-care development, facilitation and support including prescribing, health promotion and quality.
- GP fundholding promotion and development.
- Lead role on localities and locality commissioning.
- Primary-care complaints.
- Co-ordinating responsibility for issues relating to ethnic minority populations.
- Personnel, training and development for primary care and in support of corporate management.

Attached to this Directorate is also a project to provide health care and advice for single and homeless people, in both Bath and Bristol. In addition, Avon Health also has a Primary Care Audit Group in operation.

### Finance Directorate

- Financial strategy and management.
- Financial support to the Contracting Directorate.
- Primary-care support services (formerly patient data services and General Medical Services).
- Dental, pharmaceutical and ophthalmic contracts.
- Preschool child health records and information.
- Information and information technology support to all HA functions.

### Public Health Directorate

- Health needs assessment.
- Knowledge-based purchasing, effectiveness and quality.
- Clinical research, development and dissemination.
- Clinical audit.
- Lead role on strategic planning.
- Clinical advice to the HA.

## CONTRACTING DIRECTORATE

### Purchasing health services

An average HA spends approximately £300,000,000 on health services for its local population each year. On average, 95% of these services are provided by local NHS Trusts.

In order to place contracts with local NHS Trusts for the services it requires, the HA must first establish the health needs of its population, for example how many hip operations are likely to be required. The number of GP referrals and the number of hospital admissions will help inform the HA of demand. In drawing up its contract with the Trusts, the HA will also assess:

- The prevalence of particular conditions.
- Information on the effectiveness of treatment of these conditions.
- Information on where and when people want these appropriate treatments.

The HA will then consider the particular service specifications it expects the Trust to provide, such as what it would expect to provide under the accident and emergency service and the level of quality offered. There are currently thought to be a total of 56 services available through NHS Trusts and provider units, ranging from gynaecology to plastic surgery.

It is also essential for the HA to establish from the Trust how much these services are going to cost. This information is then used as the basis of the contract which the HA places with the relevant Trust or provider unit.

## Monitoring provider activity

The HA monitors the level of activity within the Trust on a monthly basis. This allows a direct comparison between the actual level of activity and the expected level specified in the contract. This information, coupled with knowledge gained through close liaison with the Trusts, is used to influence the level of contracted activity within the current year and for contracts placed in subsequent years.

If the level of activity is running consistently above contracted levels, the HA can negotiate waiting list initiatives which allow the extra activity to be carried out to help satisfy the increased demand for surgery. This extra activity can then be incorporated into a higher baseline in future contracts, to enable the HA to reflect more accurately the amount of surgery required.

## Quality of contracts with NHS Trusts

The contracts placed with NHS Trusts and other providers include a range of quality standards which incorporate the rights and standards set out in the *Patients' Charter*.

HAs receive quarterly reports from the Trusts on the quality of services they are providing, including reports on local charter standards. Some of the key areas targeted for assessment are listed in Box 2.

## Registration and inspection of nursing homes

All local private nursing homes, private treatment centres and private hospitals have to be registered with the Health Authority. Each HA has a small team of staff who inspect premises already registered, and new premises applying for registration, to ensure that they meet the requirements laid down in the *Registered Homes Act* 1984.

## CORPORATE MANAGEMENT DIRECTORATE

### Public relations

This Directorate is responsible for distributing Health Authority papers and press notices to the local media, and will take part in press, radio and TV interviews.

### Complaints

HAs monitor all complaints made to local hospitals and community services, and produce a quarterly report.

### Stores

Corporate Management is also responsible for the stores department through which most stationery and forms used at the practice are ordered. However, some forms, especially those relating to practice staff, may come directly from the Finance Directorate.

### Reception staff

All HAs will have a switchboard staffed by their own staff to take incoming calls. These staff will also deal with members of the public, GPs, dentists, opticians and pharmacists, as well as visitors from other NHS bodies who call directly at reception.

## DEVELOPMENT DIRECTORATE

### Locality purchasing

Many HAs are currently developing a basis for locality purchasing by identifying numbers of localities with an average population of 70,000; this will vary from one HA to another, and is based on groupings of GPs and their practice populations.

It is hoped that locality purchasing will enable HAs to work more closely with various groups within the local population to understand local concerns. It also allows HAs to take account of information gathered by GPs about their practice populations and, in turn, to share the information they hold about the needs of people in the district and the way they use health services.

The negotiation of contracts between the HA and the NHS Trusts will be assisted by the HA entering into discussions with GPs, local health workers and other local groups. It should also mean that HAs will be able to support GPs in their own direct discussions with hospital doctors about the ways in which they refer patients for specialist investigations and treatment. For example, one locality group has been working towards producing a protocol for neurology referrals to a particular Trust. The protocol is for patients aged between 16 and 75 years who require epileptic care.

After recent discussions with the consultant neurologist at the Trust, a revised protocol has been agreed which allows the GP direct-access service for appropriate tests.

## Maintenance of health centres

Many health centre premises, unlike hospitals and clinic buildings, have remained in Health Authority ownership. Their age and condition varies very significantly, and some of the older centres require substantial maintenance work and internal reorganisation to bring them up to modern standards.

The HA works to establish a programme of improvements to health centre premises. Funding for backlog repairs to the structure and fabric of health centres can be as high as £270,000.

HAs have contracts with NHS Trusts to maintain and service health centre buildings.

## Disposal of unused properties

Many HAs have a number of surplus NHS properties and sites within their particular area. Although NHSE Regional Offices are responsible for the marketing and sale of surplus properties, the HA meets their essential maintenance costs and other outgoings.

## Joint finance

Joint finance is a special funding allocation given to HAs to be used in ways agreed with local authorities and the voluntary sector to help develop community care. These arrangements are usually made in the Joint Consultative Committee (JCC); examples of these joint projects are:

- An interpreting service for deaf patients.
- Residential care for people with learning difficulties.
- Accommodation for recovery from drug addiction.
- Alcohol advisory schemes.

## Special projects/contracts department

This department has responsibility for the maintenance of the Authority building and any major building projects regarding the Authority headquarters it may wish to get involved in.

In Avon, it is also specifically responsible for the management of the HA's Homeless Project. This is a project for providing primary health-care services to homeless people. Under the scheme, clients can attend surgery sessions at a day centre which is staffed by a doctor and two nurses.

Its other functions include:

- Responsibility for co-ordinating the Community Needle and Exchange Scheme for people who are misusing drugs.
- Providing advice to GPs on applications to the HA's minor surgery list.
- Co-ordinating Practice Annual Reports.

## Consumer services department

The main roles of this department are:

- To ensure the accessibility of primary care by consulting the public and providing information about the services provided by contractors.
- Investigating complaints made by members of the public against any NHS services provided by a contractor.
- Liaising with Community Health Councils.
- Carrying out surveys on patient views on GP practices and GP views on the services provided by the HA.
- Designing and editing public information literature.

## Personnel and training department

As its title suggests, this department is responsible for personnel and training matters for both HA staff and GP practice staff alike.
Other functions include:

- responsibility for setting the GP practice staff training budget
- approving reimbursement of practice staff training courses
- recruitment advertising
- administering recruitment procedures.

## The Medical Adviser

The Medical Adviser is responsible for overseeing specific services relating to general medical practice. This includes encouraging rational GP prescribing and the co-ordination of health promotion. Clinical matters are also the responsibility of the Medical Adviser.

## Pharmaceutical Adviser

The Pharmaceutical Adviser generally works with the Medical Adviser, encouraging rational prescribing and the production of practice-based formularies.

## Health promotion facilitators

This area of work is broadly based around the *Health of the Nation* document, which was published in July 1992. The document sets targets for health promotion in five key areas:

1. Coronary heart disease and stroke.
2. Cancers (lung, skin, breast and cervical).
3. Accidents.
4. Mental illness.
5. HIV/AIDS and sexual health.

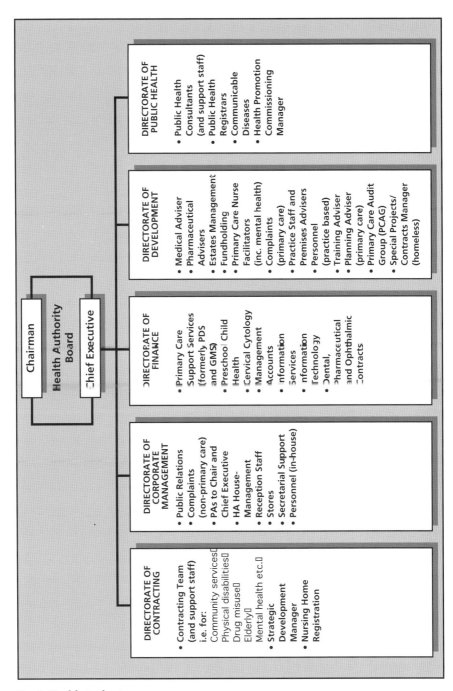

*Fig 6. Health Authority structure*

### Dietitian project

Many HAs provide funding for dietetic posts as an initiative to improve access to dietetic services by patients.

### Fundholding department

GP fundholding as a whole is discussed in greater detail in a separate section of this book (see Chapter 10). However, the fundholding department provides advice and training on accounting matters and contract negotiation.

### Practice premises/staff adviser

The key areas of responsibility associated with this post are:

- The setting of practice staff budgets for GP practices.
- The management of the HA's cost rent and improvement grant schemes (these are schemes which give financial assistance to GPs in order to assist them to build or improve their surgery premises).

## FINANCE DIRECTORATE

The Finance Directorate is responsible for the administration of contracts and payments to all four contractor groups (GPs, dentists, pharmacists and opticians). It also manages the HA's own budget for staff and running costs.

### Information services

The old Information Services Directorate has now been incorporated into the Finance Directorate and is responsible for the management of information systems and information technology.

### Primary care support services (formerly patient data services and General Medical Services [GMS])

One of the main responsibilities of this department is the provision of medical cards for patients and the subsequent transfer of medical records from one GP to another. The need for this occurs when a patient either changes address or moves area, and therefore registers with a different GP.

The department is also responsible for the quarterly capitation count of how many patients are registered with an individual GP.

Other functions include:

- Recall systems for cervical cytology and breast screening.
- Assignment of patients to a GP list.
- Applications for patients to be placed on hardship dispensing lists.
- Processing of contraceptive and registration fee claims.
- Temporary resident claim forms.
- Prescription exemption.

This department also shoulders the responsibilities of the old General Medical Services for the administration of the contracts held between the Authority and GPs. It is also responsible for processing the various claims for payment made by GPs, such as basic practice allowance, capitation fees, rent and rates reimbursement etc.

The department processes claims which are known as 'items of service'. These include:

- night visit fees
- minor surgery fees
- maternity services
- vaccinations
- contraceptive fees.

In addition, the department is also responsible for:

- administration of superannuation for GPs
- practice staff reimbursement
- trainee payments
- postgraduate education allowance (PGEA)
- doctors' deputising service.

## Information technology

This department not only maintains and supports the HA's own database and computer network, but can also be involved in such projects as the HA/GP Links Project. This project involves the electronic exchange of data between the HA and GP surgeries using the Healthlink Network. It is hoped that at least 95% of all practices will be transmitting their claims for payment by this method within the next three years.

Other functions include:

- The collation of information on outpatient and inpatient/day-case waiting times.
- The production of a series of local directories giving full details of all NHS GPs, dentists, pharmacists and opticians within the HA.
- Advising on new equipment.

## Preschool child health

This department has responsibility for the management of child health records from birth to school entry. It is also responsible for the management of the computerised child immunisation and health surveillance programmes.

## Dental, Pharmaceutical and Ophthalmic (DPO) Department

The DPO department is responsible for the administration of contracts held between the Authority and NHS dentists, pharmacists and opticians. This includes planning and payment for services carried out.

## Management Accounting Department

The Management Accounts Department is responsible for maintaining accounts and providing information as required by auditors, the DoH and the NHSE Regional Office.

## PUBLIC HEALTH DIRECTORATE

In order to deliver this health care, HAs monitor ill-health and the presence of those risk factors that are known to lead to ill-health. These risk factors include:

- long-standing illnesses and disability
- smoking
- excessive drinking
- environmental factors.

### Extra-contractual referrals (ECRs)

A small amount of the HA's budget is spent on the treatment of individual patients in hospitals with which the HA has no contracts. These are known as 'extra-contractual referrals'. These usually occur when elderly patients wish to be treated in a hospital which is close to relatives or friends who can visit and look after them. They may also occur where a particular service is required and is not provided by a local Trust, for example the treatment of children at Great Ormond Street Hospital.

Some HAs, in an attempt to curb the rise in ECRs, will refuse to fund routine referrals by GPs which duplicate those services available locally.

The exception to this will always be patients requiring emergency treatment while away from home.

### Control of infection

Although the main role of the HA is to purchase health services to meet the needs of the local population, it also has other responsibilities. Consultants in public health medicine within the HA have continued to exercise control of communicable diseases and to act as formal advisers to local district councils.

Some of the specific functions carried out by the consultants in communicable diseases are:

- The standardisation of outbreak control plans held by NHS Trusts and local authorities.
- The preparation of a unified policy for the handling and disposal of clinical waste.

Communicable diseases include:

- food poisoning
- dysentery
- meningitis
- tuberculosis (TB).

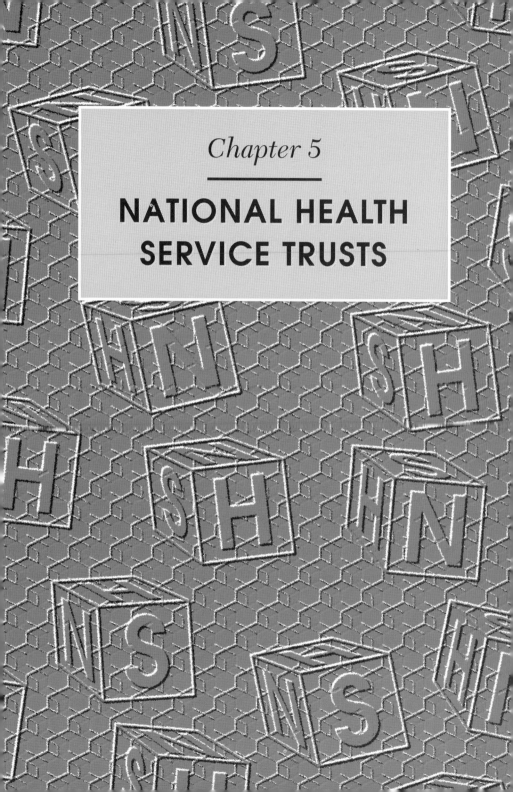

# Chapter 5

## NATIONAL HEALTH SERVICE TRUSTS

## STRUCTURE AND FUNCTION

### Background

The first wave of general hospitals granted Trust status occurred in April 1992. The majority of other hospitals have now followed in their wake.

### Main functions

In basic terms, a Trust provides a wide variety of specialist and general health services which have been purchased from it by the HA. It also provides services for other HAs from both inside and outside of its local region, and GP fund-holders.

For many Trusts, three-quarters of their resources are used to provide acute hospital services. In general, half of this income is required to provide emergency care.

### Organisation

Trust Boards meet on a monthly basis, and are accountable to the Secretary of State for strategic and policy issues, and for ensuring the delivery of national and local objectives.

The Board, as for HAs, comprises a Chairman and a number of non-executive and executive members. The Chief Executive of the Trust is also an executive member of the Board.

The Trust has a management team which is responsible for the operational management and the development of policy within the Trust. The management team is made up of the executive directors and the clinical directors of the Trust.

The clinical directors are consultant medical staff accountable to the Chief Executive for the management of patient care and treatment. This ensures the close involvement of clinical staff in the development and management of services. A large proportion of operational decisions are made close to the patient by the individual specialty or department. Clinical liaison group members comprise local GPs and the clinical directors. Professional advice is provided at committee level by representatives of the major care staff groups. The organisations which take part in joint planning are officers of social services departments, voluntary organisations and Community Health Councils (see Figure 7).

### Clinical directorates

Within each Trust, there are usually several directorates. These directorates work alongside other agencies to provide the services required; for example, the Community and Mental Health Directorate works in close association with GPs, child and family psychiatry, and mental health of elderly people.

Trusts which provide a wide range of acute medical and surgical services also have the services managed by these clinical directorates; for example,

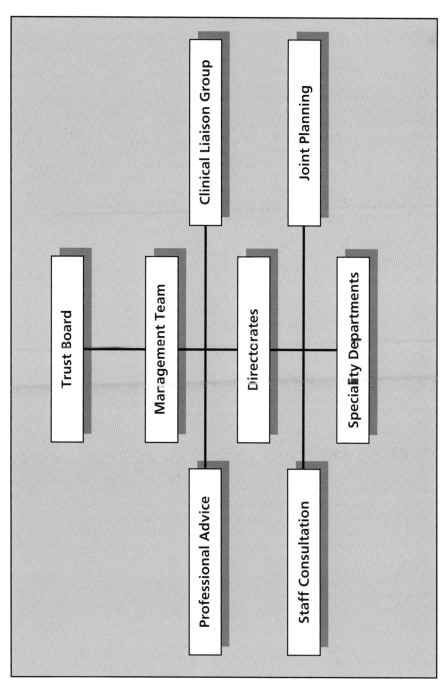

*Fig 7. NHS Trust management structure*

the clinical directorates of medicine, surgery and neurosciences.

The income generated by a Trust is used to provide and support a wide range of hospital, outpatient and community health services, details of which are given in the rest of this chapter (see Figure 8).

## MAIN SERVICES PROVIDED

### Day hospital services (for elderly people)

Many day hospitals are used for patients who need assessment, treatment and rehabilitation, but who do not need inpatient care.

Patients are referred for day hospital attendance from many sources, including outpatient clinics, physiotherapists, GPs, consultants and other health-care professionals.

The aims of day hospitals are to:

- Enable elderly people to live as independently as possible in the community.
- Rehabilitate elderly people who have been ill, or are ill, by treatment and supervision.
- Provide treatment which cannot be given at home, thus preventing or delaying admission to hospital as an inpatient.
- Enable patients to be discharged from hospital earlier than would otherwise be possible.
- Continue treatment and give advice to enable patients to maintain optimum function after discharge from hospital.
- Promote good health.

### Outpatient departments

The role of the outpatient department is to provide:

- Investigation and diagnosis, or confirmation of a GP diagnosis by a specialist.
- Follow-up treatment and supervision of the patient, if the diagnosis is confirmed.
- An accident and emergency service.

With the exception of accident and emergency (A&E), all patients seen at outpatient departments must have been referred there by a GP. This link is essential in maintaining continuity of care and the comprehensive updating of patients' records.

Each Trust will offer a variety of clinics, which may include some or all of the following:

- chest diseases
- dermatology
- ear, nose and throat (ENT)
- general medicine

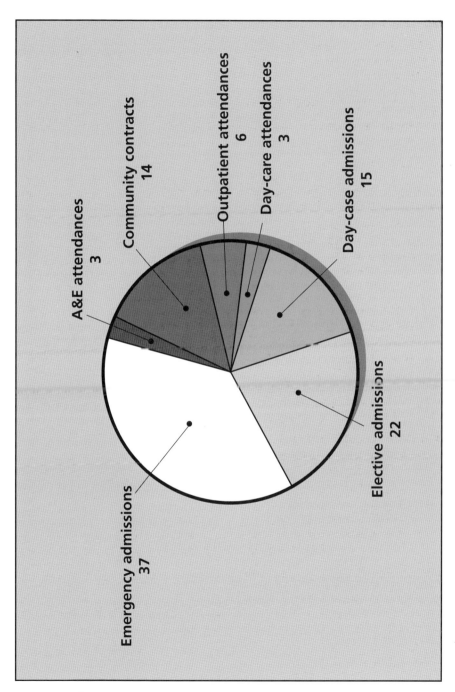

*Fig 8. Uses of NHS Trust income (%)*

- general surgery
- geriatric medicine
- gynaecology
- ophthalmics
- orthodontics
- orthopaedic surgery
- paediatrics
- rheumatology
- urology.

## Accident and emergency (A&E) departments

Organisation of this department varies from one NHS Trust/hospital to another. In some areas, it is not unusual for two hospitals to share A&E duties.

The department usually comprises a consultant, a registrar and a number of senior house officers. In addition, nurses will also be on duty as well as a number of people providing clerical support, especially on reception. A&E departments will deal with the following conditions:

- Minor injuries, such as sprains and lacerations.
- Casualties who are given instant emergency treatment and then admitted to hospital, for example heart attack, stroke, road traffic accident victims.
- Some conditions that GPs feel unable to treat and thus refer to hospital.

## X-ray departments

X-ray departments are staffed by radiologists and radiographers. Radiologists are doctors who have undertaken specialist training in the use of X-ray equipment and other methods of imaging. Radiographers are technical staff who have trained, and qualified, in the use of imaging techniques.

X-ray departments no longer merely produce standard X-rays, but now employ a number of techniques to display the internal structures of the body. The internal structures can be displayed using:
- computerised tomography
- ultrasonography
- magnetic-resonance imaging.

### Computerised tomography (CT) scanning

This is often known as 'whole body scanning'. The technique uses the X-ray process, but the data are fed into a computer and then analysed. The result is that the body can be seen in a cross-sectional manner and in greater detail.

### Ultrasound scanning

Again, this process uses the principle of analysis via cross-section. Ultrasonic waves penetrate the body, and these reflected waves are then processed by a computer to produce an image of the body. Ultrasonic scanning is particularly useful in examining pregnant women, as the sound waves are harmless to the body.

### Magnetic resonance imaging (MRI)

Here, once again, the body is analysed in cross-sectional form. MRI is mostly used to examine diseases of the central nervous system (brain and spinal cord) and the musculoskeletal system. MRI uses a powerful magnetic field to align hydrogen ions in the body fluids. The distortion of the magnetic field of the body is then analysed by a complex computer process.

### Other areas of pathology

As well as using imaging techniques to identify areas of abnormal structure within the body, it is now possible for radiologists to obtain a more accurate diagnosis by removing a small piece of tissue from the body which is then examined by a pathologist. The use of wires, tubes and catheters to perform small surgical procedures is also becoming more extensive. In the main, however, most patients are still examined by using the traditional X-ray and ultrasound methods.

## Operating theatres

Many large hospitals now have separate operating theatres. In basic terms, the work of the operating theatres covers two main areas:

- Emergency cases - these can take place at any time during the night or day.
- Non-emergency surgery - dealing with:
  a. Cases admitted from the waiting list.
  b. Cases admitted for surgery, but found to be in need of medical care before surgery.
  c. Minor surgery.

Decisions about who should receive surgery, and at what time, are taken by the surgical team and theatre staff.

## Intensive care/therapy unit (ITU)

An intensive care unit will provide a constant level of medical and nursing attention for the critically ill. Cases referred to intensive care units include patients who:

- have had major surgery
- need continuous monitoring
- need maintenance of an airway
- need control of toxaemia
- have suffered a heart attack
- have multiple, and in particular serious, head injuries.

## THERAPIES AVAILABLE

The therapy services offered by many Trusts are:

- physiotherapy
- occupational therapy
- speech and language therapy
- hearing therapy
- chiropody and foot care
- learning disabilities therapy.

The aim of each of the therapies is to improve patients' quality of life and independence through assessment, treatment, advice and education on the management of disease and disability. The promotion of health and prevention of disease is encouraged wherever possible.

All the assessments and treatments are undertaken by qualified therapists who are state registered and/or members of registered national professional organisations:

- State registered physiotherapist.
- Occupational health nurse - a qualified RGN with a post-registration qualification in occupational health nursing.
- State registered chiropodist.
- Speech therapist - member of the College of Speech and Language Therapists.
- Audiologists appear not to have a recognised qualification or associated body, but the Audiology Unit is often headed by an audiological scientist.

Each profession adheres to national professional standards and is monitored on a regular basis. The skills of all therapists are maintained by an ongoing programme of in-service training and external courses.

The aim of the therapy-services teams is to work as closely as possible with primary health-care teams (PHCTs), and increase the responsiveness of the service to GP and patient needs.

### Physiotherapy

Many Trusts have physiotherapists who have clinical expertise in treatment such as:

- mobilisation and manipulative techniques
- treatment of sports injuries
- neurological rehabilitation
- orthopaedics
- respiratory care
- obstetric and gynaecological physiotherapy.

Physiotherapy services are usually provided at outpatient departments in Trust hospitals. Practice-based physiotherapy is also available to GPs wishing to purchase an in-house service. Domiciliary physiotherapy is also available.

## Occupational therapy (OT)

Occupational therapy can help people to overcome the disabling affects of physical illness, trauma or handicap. The methods employed are based on function using purposeful activities. Conditions which can be helped include:

- arthritis
- burns
- stroke
- amputation
- hand injury
- head injury
- Parkinson's disease
- fractures
- spinal injury
- joint replacement
- surgery
- degenerative neurological conditions
- disabilities associated with ageing
- cardiac conditions.

Through evaluation and treatment, occupational therapists and occupational therapy assistants help people to:

- Learn to care for their personal needs, such as washing and dressing.
- Develop or improve the skills necessary to participate in work and leisure activities.
- Learn new ways to perform household chores, such as meal preparation, shopping and managing finances.
- Return to work and resume community activities.
- Regain the use of an injured arm, hand or leg.

Occupational therapists can also carry out wheelchair assessment and training.

## Speech and language therapy

Speech and language therapy helps children and adults to overcome communication difficulties resulting from physical, psychological or social problems.

Treatment may be given individually, in groups, or by the parent or a responsible adult (teacher or classroom assistant), working on the advice of the therapist. The treatment plan will be agreed with the patient/carer and monitored by continuous assessment.

Clinics are held in hospitals, health centres, special schools and units throughout a Trust.

## Hearing therapy

Hearing therapy is a rehabilitation service for the hearing impaired, who may have sensory neural hearing loss, conductive hearing loss, tinnitus, hyperacusis or obscure auditory dysfunction. The service is either delivered in a group forum or on an individual basis, and provides an opportunity for counselling on the long-term implications of the condition. The hearing therapy service offers:

- An assessment of the patient's condition.
- Provision of information about hearing aids, environmental aids and other communication appliances.
- Training in the development and use of communication skills such as speech reading, hearing tactics and listening skills.
- Therapeutic treatments, such as relaxation therapy, tinnitus management, management of balance disorders, and support of cochlear implant users.

Many Trusts have a hearing therapy volunteer scheme which offers a domiciliary service to first-time hearing-aid users over the age of 60.

## Chiropody and footcare

Chiropody and footcare is usually delivered from clinics located throughout the locality. A limited domiciliary service may be available for housebound patients. The scope of chiropody and footcare includes:

- corns
- calluses
- plantar warts
- nail pathologies
- ulceration
- infection
- biomechanical evaluation (assessment of the degree of movement within the joints and the steps taken to correct it)
- nail surgery under local anaesthetic.

Patients can self-refer or be referred by the primary health-care team or a consultant. The first consultation is with a State Registered Chiropodist, who formulates a treatment plan. Many patients require ongoing routine care.

Residential and nursing homes may arrange a domiciliary footcare and chiropody service with the Trust, which will entail qualified chiropodists and assistants visiting the home at agreed intervals. Training in basic footcare for staff of the home can also be provided.

## Learning disabilities

The aim of this service is to increase the independence of adults with learning disabilities by using a variety of specialist techniques. Therapists work in multi-agency community teams in partnership with social workers, clinical psychologists and the voluntary sector. Services include:

- speech and language therapy
- community nursing
- specialist clinical nursing (challenging behaviour)
- occupational therapy
- physiotherapy.

## OTHER SERVICES

Specialties such as rheumatology and dermatology are also provided for local residents.

Pathology, and A&E operating theatres are managed by clinical support and clinical directorates. Obviously, not every Trust will provide all the services detailed above; or these services may be provided by Trusts on an individual basis within the locality.

The majority of community services, such as district nursing and health visiting, are provided for local residents from a network of health centres, clinics and community health team bases.

## NON-CLINICAL DIRECTORATES

As well as the clinical directorates, a Trust will also contain a number of non-clinical directorates, such as finance, estates, information and personnel.

As previously stated, NHS Trusts work closely with social services, voluntary organisations and Community Health Councils in planning the provision of their services.

## Patients' representatives

A few Trusts have appointed a patients' representative, whose chief role is to take the concerns and wishes of patients into account. These posts are funded by the National Association of Health Authorities and Trusts (NAHAT). The main aims of NAHAT are listed in Box 3.

## Clinical liaison groups

These have been established since 1992, and provide a regular forum for direct communication between local GPs and the clinical directors of the Trust.

## BOX 3 THE MAIN AIMS OF THE NATIONAL ASSOCIATION OF HEALTH AUTHORITIES AND TRUSTS

To investigate and give voice to specific problems of concern to its membership.

•

To foster co-operation and communication between NHS authorities, NHS Trusts, government departments, local authorities and other organisations concerned with health matters.

•

To educate and inform the public about the achievements and needs of the NHS.

•

To promote research, education and the exchange of information within the NHS.

•

To advise government and professional bodies on issues relating to the NHS.

# Chapter 6

## NHS SERVICES

# AMBULANCE SERVICES

In theory, the Secretary of State has responsibility for providing ambulance services to meet the needs of the population. In reality, this role is delegated to nominated NHS authorities.

At present there are 55 ambulance services in England, Wales and Northern Ireland, and a national unitary service in Scotland.

Since 1990, ambulance services have tendered for contracts to provide services. A number have in fact become NHS Trusts. Recently there has been a distinct split between the emergency and urgent services, and non-urgent services provided.

## Emergency and urgent ambulance services

Purchasing authorities are required to place contracts for the provision of emergency and ambulance services for the practice population they cover.

The ambulance service must respond to the following:

- 999 calls.
- Doctors' urgent admissions.
- Urgent interhospital transfers and high dependency transfers.
- Major incidents (ambulance services must have plans to respond to such emergencies as airport disasters etc).

The staff of ambulances responding to accident and emergency calls must have completed the NHS Training Directorate's basic course or obtained the relevant National Vocational Qualification (NVQ).

The *Patients' Charter* is used to define performance standards specified in contracts for ambulance services, and includes the following as a minimum:

- In 50% of all emergency calls, an ambulance will be with the patient within eight minutes.
- In 95% of all emergency calls, an ambulance will reach the patient within 14 minutes in urban areas and 19 minutes in rural areas.
- In 95% of all urgent calls from clinicians, the patient will reach the treatment centre within 15 minutes of the agreed time.

Ambulance services are also often asked to attend sporting activities and other public events.

## Non-emergency patient services

This service involves the transportation of patients who, while requiring treatment, do not require an immediate response. It should also allow them to reach hospital in a reasonable time and in reasonable comfort.

This can involve the use of hospital cars driven by volunteers, or ambulances designed to function more in the role of minibuses.

## Paramedics

Each emergency and urgent ambulance has a paramedic on board. The main role of the paramedic is to stabilise the patient before arrival at the hospital.

## BLOOD TRANSFUSION SERVICES

Since 1993, the management of all NHS blood services has been carried out by a single body. The National Blood Authority (NBA) also has a responsibility for all Regional Transfusion Centres (RTCs). From 1995 the NBA has been organised into three zonal centres which have been established in Bristol, Leeds and North London. Bulk processing and testing have thus been transferred away from other regional centres to these three areas. In addition, it is hoped that an additional two blood banks will be added to the existing network of 15 which supplies blood to hospitals. The key objectives of the National Blood Authority are shown in Box 4.

---

### BOX 4 *THE MAIN OBJECTIVES OF THE NATIONAL BLOOD AUTHORITY*

To maintain and promote blood, and blood product, supply based on the system of voluntary donors.

•

To implement a cost-effective national strategy for ensuring an adequate supply of blood and blood products to meet national needs.

•

To ensure that high standards of safety and quality are maintained throughout the blood service.

•

To ensure the cost-efficient operation of the transfusion centres and International Blood Group Reference Laboratory as parts of the national service.

---

All RTCs collect blood and prepare blood products. The use of plasma, the fluid in which the components of blood are suspended, rather than whole blood itself, is increasing. So is the use of the cellular components such as red cells and platelets. RTCs also perform specialist services, such as tissue typing for organ and bone marrow transplants.

The blood transfusion service is completely dependent on voluntary donors. It is the role of the RTC to ascertain the blood group of the donor, and then to ensure that the blood is safe and does not contain any infectious agents.

Hospitals reimburse the RTCs according to the service and products they use.

## CHILD HEALTH SERVICES

### Professionals involved

Child health services is a term used to cover the wide area of work associated with babies, children and adolescents (those under 16 years old). The care for this group is provided by professionals both in the community and in hospital. The doctors one would usually expect to provide child health services are GPs, hospital specialists, paediatricians and surgical specialists.

### Community paediatricians

This area of work involves caring for the needs of the entire child population in a particular locality. Community paediatricians are usually based at health centres and associated clinics, and provide services to children in the following areas:

- school health
- children in care
- children with special needs.

### Ethnic minorities

It has been well established that children from minority ethnic groups have special health-care needs. For example, one in every 400 West Indian babies will have sickle-cell anaemia, while disorders such as rickets and anaemia are prevalent among Asian children.

### Vaccinations

Babies are currently immunised at two, three and four months. Vaccinations carried out over this period of time will be for polio, diphtheria, tetanus and pertussis (whooping cough). MMR (mumps, measles and rubella) is given when a child is between 12-15 months old. In addition, all children have a pre-school booster at 4-4½ years old.

Children are also often vaccinated against *Haemophilus influenzae* B (Hib), which is thought to be associated with meningitis.

In March 1996, children and young people were given their own *Patients' Charter*.

### Child health surveillance

A midwife is responsible for the mother and baby until 10 days after the baby has been born. Responsibility will then pass to a health visitor.

The health visitor will visit the mother and baby at home within a short time of them being discharged from hospital, or of a home birth, to see how both are progressing. If it appears that there may be particular problems, the health visitor may arrange to visit. The frequency of these visits depends upon local Trust policy and the particular circumstances involved. In an abuse case, a health visitor could be visiting on a daily basis.

As the baby develops, it is more usual for mothers to travel to child health clinics to have their babies checked by health visitors and GPs to see that they are developing normally.

Recently it has become more usual for GPs to become involved in child health surveillance programmes. Indeed, they receive payment from the HA for such work, providing that they are suitably qualified and on the HA's register. The screening of children takes place at the following predetermined intervals:

- neonatal
- 6-8 weeks
- 6-9 months
- 18-24 months
- 3-4 years (preschool).

## Hospitalisation

Where possible, children are nursed in designated children's ward. Facilities should also be available for the parents of the child, for example a place to sleep. The Department of Health requires that at least two registered 'sick children's nurses' should be on duty at any one time; this standard, however, is often not met. It is also preferred that surgical operations are carried out by surgeons and anaesthetists who are used to dealing with children on a regular basis.

## The *Children Act*

This particular Act came into force in October 1991. The main bulk of the document deals with the courts and the social services departments.

However, there are several which have a direct affect on Health Authorities, especially where they are negotiating the levels and types of service provision with social services.

It is stated that HAs and Trusts should take into account:

- The duty to collaborate with social services departments in providing the services to support children in need and their families.
- The duty to inform the responsible social services department when a Health Authority or Trust intends to provide accommodation for a child for a consecutive period of three months, and when such a child leaves the accommodation.

- The duty to apply the Children (Secure Accommodation) Regulations 1991 to children whose liberty is restricted in an NHS establishment other than under *Mental Health Act* provisions.

## LABORATORY SERVICES

An increasing number of GPs now send blood, body tissues and fluids to pathology departments for analysis. However, most pathology work still stems from hospital referrals. Pathology departments are usually divided into four major sections:

a) Clinical chemistry.

b) Haematology.

c) Histopathology.

d) Microbiology.

### Clinical chemistry

Clinical chemistry is based around an analytical and advisory/interpretative service for a range of analyses concerned with body fluids and tissues.

The role of the clinical chemist is to advise on how to use the service, how to interpret the results, and the need for further investigation. Advice is often given in the areas of management of diabetes, management of lipid disorders, and therapeutic drug monitoring. A great many of the tests are processed automatically, for example chemical tests for renal and liver diseases. A large number of specialist tests cannot be automated. Monitoring of drug therapy is such as example.

### Haematology

Haematology laboratory services can be divided into three sections:

a) Investigation of blood cells and their abnormalities, e.g. leukaemia or anaemia.

b) Investigation of bleeding and clotting disorders, e.g. thrombosis, haemophilia.

c) Blood transfusion.

A close link between the regional transfusion centres and the hospital 'blood banks' is maintained at all times. The haematology laboratory is responsible for supporting patients undergoing bone-marrow transplants and chemotherapy for leukaemia.

### Histopathology

This concerns the examination of tissues in the cells. Most cervical cytology screening is also carried out in histopathology laboratories. In addition to providing a diagnostic service, most laboratories also undertake postmortem examinations.

## Microbiology

Microbiology laboratories are chiefly concerned with examining specimens from patients for bacteria, fungi and viruses. They also screen food and environmental samples for microbiological contamination.

Microbiology is also involved in the control of infection in hospital wards, kitchens and operating theatres.

## MATERNITY SERVICES

Maternity services require a co-ordinated approach from GPs, midwives, obstetricians, paediatricians, health visitors and, in some cases, social and link workers.

### GPs

Many GPs provide a complete package of maternity care in conjunction with the midwifery service.

### Midwives

Midwives are employed to supervise, advise and care for women during pregnancy and a 'normal' childbirth. In an abnormal birth they will also support obstetricians. Midwives work in the community with GPs and in hospital with obstetricians.

### Obstetricians

Obstetricians are usually involved with high-risk pregnancies and when emergencies occur. An expectant mother is usually under the care of an obstetrician, but when visiting the hospital, for example for a scan, if the pregnancy is normal she is more likely to see a radiographer than the obstetrician.

### Antenatal care

Antenatal care should be locally available to all pregnant women. It usually combines a mixture of GP/clinic-based care and some additional hospital input. Some patients prefer all hospital care.

### Postnatal care

The following are paramount to good postnatal care:

- Uniform and consistent advice on infant feeding including promotion of, and support for, breast feeding.
- The length of postnatal hospital stay, based on the mother's and the baby's health and social needs.
- Adequate facilities in hospital for privacy and the establishment of parenting.
- A full range of professional advice.
- Clear hand-over arrangements between the hospital and the community.

In addition, clear guidelines should be in place for dealing with the death of babies, babies who are handicapped and admitted to special baby care units, and those who are adopted, fostered or taken into care.

Major government initiatives on maternity services have included:

- The establishment of an expert maternity group - this led to the publication of the document *Changing Childbirth*. This document included such recommendations as the right of women to choose who cares for them during pregnancy and childbirth, and the right to choose the type of care wanted.
- The establishment of a maternity services task force led by the NHS Executive to examine and disseminate good practice in selected aspects of the management of the service.
- A Department of Health/NHS Maternity Unit Study Team to examine examples of good practice in the provision of care in units led by GPs and/or midwives.

## MENTAL HEALTH SERVICES

Mental health problems are extremely diverse, and can range from a particular life crisis to those people who suffer from dementia or schizophrenia.

Until the 1970s, most psychiatric services were provided from large mental hospitals. Currently, 60% of NHS mental hospital beds are still provided in large institutions. However, it is hoped that this number will be greatly reduced within the next six years. Most of these patients will transfer to community settings.

However, it is reasonable to assume that approximately 15% of the population will still require some form of hospital-based service.

The most recent trend has been to focus on non-hospital, multidisciplinary locality-based treatment settings. For information purposes, a multidisciplinary team will usually comprise psychiatrists, community psychiatric nurses (CPNs), occupational therapists, psychologists and social workers.

Where mental health services are still provided in a hospital setting, attempts have been made to provide a more domestic and user-friendly environment.

### Mental Health Act Commission

1983 saw the establishment of the Mental Health Act Commission, consisting of some 90 members. The majority of these members are lawyers, doctors, social workers, psychologists, lay persons and other specialists. The key functions of the commission are listed in Box 5.

## NURSING SERVICES

The largest professional group within the NHS is made up of nurses and midwives. This group includes a number of unqualified staff who are known as

## BOX 5 THE KEY FUNCTIONS OF THE MENTAL HEALTH ACT COMMISSION

To keep under review the operation of the Mental Health Act 1983 in respect of patients liable to be detained under the Act.

•

To visit and interview private patients detained under the Act, in hospitals and homes for the mentally infirm.

•

To investigate complaints which fall within the Commission's remit.

•

To review decisions to withhold the mail of patients detained in special hospitals.

•

To appoint medical practitioners and others who give second opinions in cases where this is required by the Act.

•

To publish and lay before Parliament a report every two years. (The 1991-93 report covered the five key areas of statutory functions, Commission operations, policy matters, The Mental Health Act Commission 10 years on, and other activities.)

•

To monitor the implementation of the code of practice and propose amendments to ministers.

•

To offer advice to ministers on matters falling within the Commission's remit.

health-care assistants, nursing assistants or nursing auxiliaries. Interestingly, 10% of nursing staff are men. The percentage however is much higher for psychiatric care.

The different nurses who make up this body are as follows.

### Registered nurse (RN)

A registered nurse is someone who has qualified for the first part of the nursing register (See also Chapter 8, Primary Health-Care Team Nurses). Registered nurses may be referred to as State Registered Nurse (SRN), Registered General Nurse (RGN) or Registered Nurse (RN). These are all the same qualification; before 1985 all registered nurses were known as SRNs, now RGN and RN are the common terms.

## Enrolled nurse (EN)

The training of enrolled nurses has now been phased out, but there are still many ENs still working in primary health care.

## Midwives

As with other registered nurses, midwives are viewed as being practitioners in their own right. They can also administer certain specified drugs on their own authority.

## Health visitors

These are fully trained nurses who concentrate on child health, although some have specialist roles, such as working with handicapped children or elderly people.

## Nurse practitioners

Nurse practitioners are qualified nurses who have taken an advanced course pitched at degree level. They are able to diagnose, prescribe treatment and make patient referrals. A nurse practitioner has sole responsibility for his/her actions. The term 'nurse practitioner' currently applies to approximately 200 nurses who have completed recognised courses run by the Royal College of Nursing (RCN).

Although patients may choose to see nurse practitioners when they visit a GP practice, they are always free to consult with a GP if they so prefer.

Nurse practitioners are currently employed in the following areas:

- A&E departments
- homeless centres
- women's aid refuges
- health centres
- general practices.

## Ward sister/charge nurse

Generally a ward sister is a woman, and a charge nurse is a man. They are responsible for organising and running a ward or department. Other main functions include:

- Recruitment and teaching of trained staff, nursing students and health-care assistants.
- Maintaining the correct skill and grade mix.
- Control of the budget for clinical materials.

In addition to these responsibilities, ward sisters/charge nurses also nurse patients themselves and offer support to relatives, directors and associated health-care professionals.

## Statutory bodies

The nursing profession in the UK is regulated by the United Kingdom Central Council (UKCC) for Nursing, Midwifery and Health Visiting.

The UKCC has total responsibility for monitoring a single professional register for all nurses, midwives and health visitors, and general policies on professional education and development. It also has responsibility for professional conduct.

## Primary nursing

This is a style of nursing where an identified nurse takes personal responsibility for the care of individual patients. An example of this may be during a stay in hospital, where a named nurse will have direct responsibility for a particular patient.

## Community nursing contracts

A major impact on the organisation of community nursing, and the link between acute hospital nursing and the community, has been the 1990 *National Health Service Act.*

Health Authorities now have to specify what community nursing services they need in the form of a contract. In effect, this means that nurses have to submit tenders for their services. In some cases this has resulted in awards to manage contracts being placed outside of the immediate locality; for example, nursing services in Somerset are managed by Cornwall and the Isles of Scilly.

## Nurse prescribing

Certain community nurses are allowed to prescribe a specified number of dressings and products. At the time of writing, this scheme was being piloted; it is proposed that there will be a greater number of participants in the scheme in the future.

## Project 2000

Project 2000 courses are three years long and provide a registered nursing qualification at diploma level. For 80% of their time the students are counted as being supernumerary and, while in the hospital or community setting, are not counted as part of the staff. It is hoped that this gives them more time for learning and ensures that they are not left in sole charge of the patients.

Project 2000 students are not counted as employees, and receive a bursary. The course starts with a foundation programme lasting 18 months, followed by a further 18 months in a particular branch of nursing, such as the care of adults, children, people with learning disabilities and mental health patients.

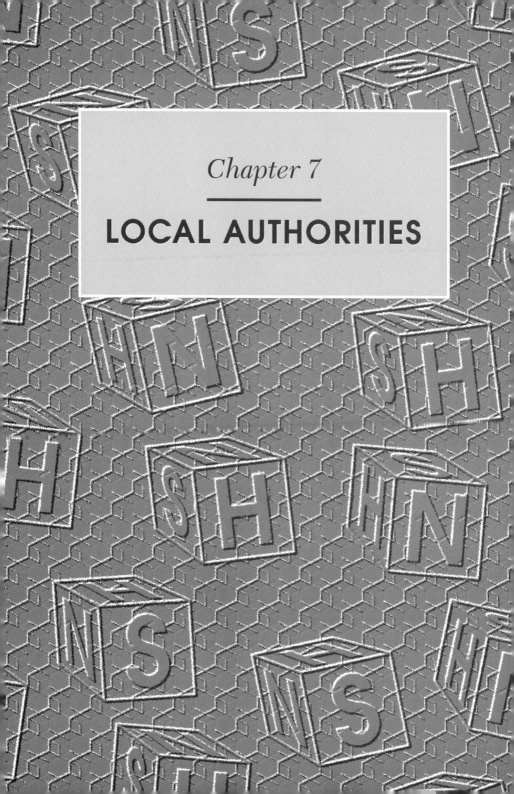

*Chapter 7*

# LOCAL AUTHORITIES

Local authorities have switched from being a two-teir system, consisting of the County Council and the District Council, to a single unitary authority. They have responsibility for all social services and public health services.

Decisions and policies implemented by local authorities are deemed to have a democratic basis, as they have been passed by various committees which comprise locally elected councillors. Before a policy has been adopted, it is possible that some of the councillors involved on the committee have been lobbied by members of the public and, in fact, a policy may be rejected at committee level.

## SOCIAL SERVICES DEPARTMENTS

The work of social services can be divided in to two distinct areas: children and adults.

The work of social services with children involves caring for those children who can be termed vulnerable, and therefore includes such issues as child protection, looking after children with impairments, fostering and adoption.

The work with adults includes caring and providing services for people with learning difficulties, elderly people and people with mental health problems and physical impairments (such as vision and hearing difficulties). In addition, social services also provide a service for those misusing alcohol and/or drugs, and for those suffering from HIV/AIDS.

### Social workers

Social workers are usually graduates who have then had one year's training in social work.

### Organisation

Social services are provided from a headquarters unit which is managed by a director and a number of assistant directors. The work is split into two areas:

### Strategy

This includes areas of responsibility such as planning, research and development, commissioning and the placing of contracts.

### Operations

This is the department actually responsible for running all the services provided. The workload will be split between a number of areas within a particular county.

The day-to-day work is carried out by social workers working within local hospital units and in teams in the community.

In addition to the main directorates of operations and strategy, the work of social services also covers the following areas:

### Inspection units

These units are responsible for the inspection of residential nursing homes, day nurseries and registered childminders.

### Emergency duty team

This team is responsible for all out-of-hours work, such as nights and weekends, and is chiefly called upon for compulsory hospital admissions.

The work of social services is governed by a series of Acts, such as:- *The Children Act* 1989, *The Mental Health Act* 1983 and *The NHS and Community Care Act 1990.* The fact that their work is decentralised means that variations in the way services are developed and delivered can be achieved not only from county to county, but also from area to area within that county.

## FUNDING

The funding (grant) that local authorities receive depends upon central government's assessment. In effect, this means that funds are raised by direct taxation of the public.

Many local authorities are capped, and consequently receive no additional funding from year to year, although it can be argued that the cost of providing care in the community rises annually. This has led to many local authorities reporting that they have had to cut services.

In 1993/4, the Government gave a Special Transitional Grant (STG) to each social services authority to provide resources for the new community care responsibility. Even with this additional allowance, many authorities will still receive less than they require to support the numbers receiving public funding towards care costs.

At the moment, the social services department receives three specific grants which are ring-fenced:

a) Mental health.

b) Alcohol and drugs.

c) HIV/AIDS.

Although this ring-fencing is not permanent, it is unlikely to change in the near future.

### Purchasers/providers

As with many other areas within this book, there is a split between the purchasers and providers of community care (see Box 6).

However, it is important to note that the social services department has a corporate approach to arranging services, and does not like NHS bodies having separate purchaser and provider units.

## FUNCTIONS

As previously mentioned, the work of social services revolves around the key areas of children and adults. I have, therefore, detailed below some of the specific areas for which they have a direct responsibility.

## BOX 6 PURCHASERS AND PROVIDERS OF COMMUNITY CARE

Purchasers:

Social services departments.

•

Health Authorities.

•

GP fundholders.

•

Housing authorities.

Providers:

Social services departments.

•

NHS Trusts.

•

Housing authorities.

•

Voluntary organisations.

•

Other independent sector organisations.

### Play groups

The *Children Act* 1989 protects young children and ensures that certain standards are provided. It makes the registration of play groups with the local authority compulsory. Social services officers will generally visit a play group before it applies for registration to offer advice. Once a play group has been accepted for registration, the department will also carry out a minimum annual inspection.

### Register of disabled children

Social services, in conjunction with HAs and education departments, are responsible for setting up and maintaining a register of disabled children. The purpose of this register is to:

- Make sure that all children who are registered are assessed for services, and ensure that regular reviews are undertaken throughout childhood.
- Provide information on where disabled children are living and what their needs are, enabling the planning of future services to meet the needs of all disabled children within a particular county.

- Provide useful information to the parents and/or carers of children who are registered.

The register is usually held on the child-health computer system, which is managed by the HA.

All children who are placed on the register have been assessed by a community paediatrician.

## Visually impaired people

Many people whose eyesight is poor are registered with the social services department as partially sighted or blind.

A social worker will usually be in contact with the person, and will give help and advice on the services which they may be entitled to (for example talking books and magazines, reduced TV licence fee, rail fares, bus fares and parking concessions).

## Working with other agencies

This often involves working closely with voluntary agencies, such as:

| | |
|---|---|
| *Aled Richards Trust* | A voluntary organisation which provides support and care to people who are affected with HIV/AIDS. This includes counselling, health promotion, a telephone help-line etc, and is open to friends, relatives and carers of the patients. |
| *Alcoholics Anonymous* | Providing local counselling for people who wish to achieve and maintain sobriety. |
| *Cyrenians* | A charitable organisation which provides limited accommodation for people who are vulnerable, such as the homeless. In addition, the organisation also runs day centres for homeless people. |

These agencies can provide:

- Information, assessment and counselling for people concerned about their own or someone else's drinking problem.
- Information, education and advice on alcohol and its effects.
- Detoxification.
- Supervised drug consumption on a daily basis.
- Advice to professionals, family members or others regarding management of drug problems.
- Practical and emotional support for those suffering from HIV/AIDS by a specialist team of social workers and home support workers.

Most of the services are available for men and women of all ages. In addition, most counselling services are provided free of charge. Most people can make use of these services by visiting or telephoning any of the specialist agencies. Alternatively, direct referrals are sometimes made by GPs, health visitors, social workers, youth workers and probation officers.

## Community care

The main aim of community care is to enable people who need assistance in looking after themselves, to survive in their own homes. If, however, they are unable, or become unable, to do so, accommodation should be arranged for them in a residential nursing home.

The main groups of people eligible for community care are:

- Disabled people with severe and permanent impairments, who are dependent on others for any activities of daily living.
- People in receipt of, or who may be eligible for, attendance, mobility (disability living) or severe disability allowances.
- People who are terminally ill and who are, or are likely to become, highly dependent.
- People living with HIV/AIDS who have reached the stage where considerable help is needed.
- People living with any condition or impairment, including short-term sickness, which requires help to avoid risk to the safety of the individual, or the carer(s).
- People whose needs may possibly require residential or nursing home care.
- Seriously mentally-ill people and those people recovering from mental illness.
- People who are confused.
- People who require help as a result of their misuse of drugs or alcohol.
- People looking after someone, who need support to continue caring for them.

## ENVIRONMENTAL HEALTH

Public health inspectors are appointed by local authorities to carry out such duties as the inspection of shops and slaughter-houses, the regulation of markets and the inspection of food, and deal with the problem of housing where it constitutes a danger to health such as:

- infestation
- smoke
- noise nuisance.

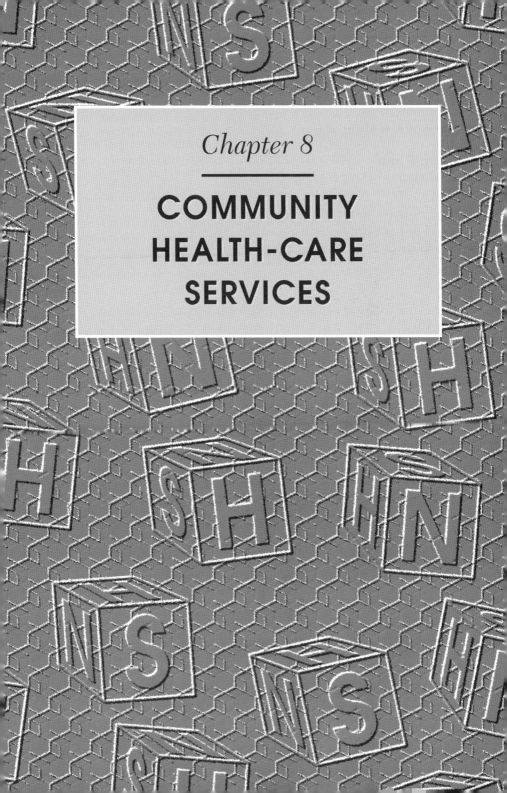

*Chapter 8*

# COMMUNITY
# HEALTH-CARE
# SERVICES

## PRIMARY HEALTH-CARE TEAM (PHCT)

Primary health care is the term used to describe the delivery of health care in a community setting. Care is delivered through the services of health-care professionals working alongside other specialist staff, such as social workers, counsellors, chiropodists and dietitians.

### Structure and main functions

The primary health-care team (PHCT) includes those professionals with whom members of the public may have their first point of contact within the health service:

- general practitioners
- practice nurses
- health visitors
- district nurses
- midwives
- practice managers
- reception staff.

The PHCT is a difficult body to define, as it tends to vary depending on the commitment to, and an individual GP's (or group of GPs') perception of, what a primary health-care team should be. In some practices, the GPs involved may only see the team as comprising themselves and the practice nurses, while other GPs see the primary health-care team as being further reaching.

It is the aim of the PHCT to work collaboratively with other members of the team, to make use of other professionals' expertise appropriately and to ensure continuity of care while preserving confidentiality.

Currently, the management of the various members of the PHCT is split. Community services are administered through the district units and Trusts, while GPs are contracted by the HA to provide medical services to patients registered with them in the community. Practice nurses are usually directly employed and managed by GPs.

### Primary health-care team nurses

*Practice nurse*

The practice nurse is usually a Registered General Nurse (RGN), but could be an Enrolled Nurse (EN), who is employed by a GP to work within the practice, often combining practical duties in the treatment room with a health promotion role. Some nurses, if appropriately qualified, may visit patients in their own home, according to agreed protocols.

Since the implementation of the GP Contract in April 1990, there has been a considerable increase in both the number of nurses employed and the range of activities in which they are involved.

### Community nursing sister (district nurse)

The district nurse is a RGN holding a District Nursing Certificate, who is employed to provide skilled nursing care for patients in the home. He or she is the nurse qualified and accountable for assessing and evaluating the nursing care of such patients.

### District enrolled nurse

These are generally now few and far between, but the district enrolled nurse is a member of the district nursing team. They are accountable to the district nurse for carrying out part, or all, of the nursing care programme for individual patients and their families. They must record their findings and report back to the district nurse.

### Health visitor

The health visitor is a RGN who has undertaken a further year of study at an institute of higher or further education to qualify for the title. He/she specialises in the promotion of health and prevention of ill-health, and may work with all members of a family including elderly people, but is mainly involved with women and young children. Some health visitors undertake other health promotion activities, such as running smoking cessation or stress management groups.

### Midwives

The midwife is a RGN who has undertaken further training to become a registered midwife. Working in the community, he/she offers a specialised service to women during all stages of pregnancy and childbirth, and has responsibility for both mother and child for 28 days following the delivery. The midwife is the only nurse qualified to undertake antenatal care.

### Other specialist nurses

There are also some specialist nurses who work within, or liaise with, the community team. These can include:

- school nurse
- diabetic liaison nurse
- paediatric nurse
- community psychiatric nurse
- stoma-care nurse
- incontinence adviser
- geriatric nurse
- treatment room nurse
- HIV liaison nurse
- breast-care adviser.

### Practice nurse trainers

Practice nurses often work closely with practice nurse trainers who provide specialist training and advice.

## HOSPICE CARE

Hospices provide services for people who are terminally ill. In addition to employing medical and nursing staff, most hospices will also employ the following:

- specialist social workers
- physiotherapists
- occupational therapists
- bereavement counsellors
- chaplains/ministers of various denominations.

There will also be a large number of volunteers working in close association, and providing a supporting role that is crucial in hospice care.

Hospices usually care for people with cancer, although more recently this role has expanded. It is a sobering thought that one in three of the population will develop cancer, and indeed one in five will actually die of it.

As previously mentioned, the role of hospices is expanding and many now care for AIDS sufferers and patients with motor neurone diseases.

There are known to be approximately 3,000 inpatient hospice beds in the UK. Four-fifths of these are in voluntary hospices and one-fifth in NHS hospice units. There are approximately 125 independent voluntary inpatient hospices, 11 Marie Curie homes and nine Sue Ryder Foundation homes. The Cancer Relief MacMillan Fund (CRMF), which also has a high profile with regard to caring for the terminally ill, usually offers care at home.

There are 50 NHS hospices, although not all their costs are always funded by the NHS and many units now have to embark on fund-raising events and rely on support through the League of Friends.

In addition, some privately owned nursing homes also offer care to the terminally ill.

There are currently approximately 200 day hospices in operation. Day hospices offer a wide range of services to patients, including:

- counselling
- chiropody
- hairdressing.

Of the 400 nursing teams caring for patients at home, most are initially funded by the Cancer Relief MacMillan Fund. The CRMF covers the cost of nursing for the first three years, after which the Health Authority takes over the funding.

Working alongside the MacMillan nurses and other home-care nurses are approximately 5,000 part-time Marie Curie nurses. These posts are funded jointly between the Health Authorities and Marie Curie Cancer Care.

Care of the terminally ill is also carried out in approximately 200 acute hospitals.

The funding for hospice care comes from the NHSE. It is hoped that Health Authorities will be able to match the same amount of funding as received from the voluntary sector.

## COMMUNITY HEALTH COUNCILS (CHCs)

The CHC is the public's so-called 'independent watchdog' for the NHS.

Its aim is to seek the best possible health care for its local population by offering free help and advice, and by influencing bodies involved in the purchasing and delivering of health care.

CHCs are funded from a national budget held by the NHSE. CHC staff are employed by Health Autorities.

### Organisation

CHC officers are members of the local community. Members of the CHC are appointed for a period of four years. In turn, half of the members are subject to reappointment every two years. In general, CHC members are employed on a voluntary basis.

Each CHC generally comprises 18-24 members. Membership of the CHC includes a chairman and a secretary. Most CHCs have at least one additional member of staff, and often part-time and research workers are employed.

CHCs will hold meetings at least once every three months, and will publish an annual report which is available to the public. Key functions of the CHCs are given in Box 7.

The CHCs' key areas of interest are examined in the form of a number of groups, examples of which are given below.

### Hospital care group

The main remit of this group is to consider and evaluate the extensive area of work carried out by NHS hospitals. CHCs have the power to enter and inspect premises owned by HAs and NHS Trusts.

To this end, the group may spend time considering concerns relating to specific services, such as the availability of paediatric intensive therapy care units and special baby care unit service.

Members of the group also undertake hospital visits over the whole district.

### Primary health- and community-care group

In terms of primary health care, this group liaises closely with HAs and the practitioners in contract to it, i.e. GPs, dentists, pharmacists and opticians. For example, CHCs may have direct discussion with the HA regarding GP patient satisfaction surveys.

## BOX 7 KEY FUNCTIONS OF THE COMMUNITY HEALTH COUNCILS

Publicising and discussing Health Authority plans and consultation documents.

•

Meeting regularly with the Health Authority.

•

Visiting hospitals and clinics to speak to patients and staff.

•

Offering free advice and information.

•

Holding regular public meetings.

•

Helping people who wish to make complaints.

•

Working in partnership with voluntary organisations and community groups.

With regard to services such as mental health and the care of the elderly, dialogue will occur between the CHC, the community and hospitals.

### Users' forums

As part of the CHC's remit to share information and listen to the concerns of people representing voluntary groups, the users' forum meets regularly with groups such as 'women and children's health' and the 'deaf women's health project', and forums on racial equality, maternity liaison and learning difficulties.

### Purchaser group

This group attempts to influence the quality and quantity of the health care which has been purchased by the HA and provided by local NHS Trusts.

### Complaints

An important part of the work of the CHC is the assistance and advice it gives to patients if they wish to make a complaint against a health professional or any other associated aspect of health care.

It is not unusual for a CHC to handle as many as 211 complaints in an individual year.

## VOLUNTARY GROUPS

Voluntary organisations provide services for the public, offer information and advice, and may represent a client group or specific issue.

All voluntary groups can be seen as offering a vital complementary service to mainstream NHS care. Examples of high-profile voluntary groups are:

**MIND**     National Association for Mental Health.

**RNID**     (Royal National Institute for the Deaf) - organisation for deaf people.

**RNIB**     (Royal National Institute for the Blind) - organisation for blind/partially-sighted people.

**Samaritans**     offering a 24-hour confidential service for people in despair and who may be suicidal.

Most of these voluntary organisations are part of the National Council for Voluntary Organisations.

Because many of these agencies are experts in the advice and services they offer, many provider units actively make use of this knowledge and in effect use them as sub-contractors. For example, some AIDS counselling may be carried out by voluntary organisations, but is in fact paid for by the local NHS Trust.

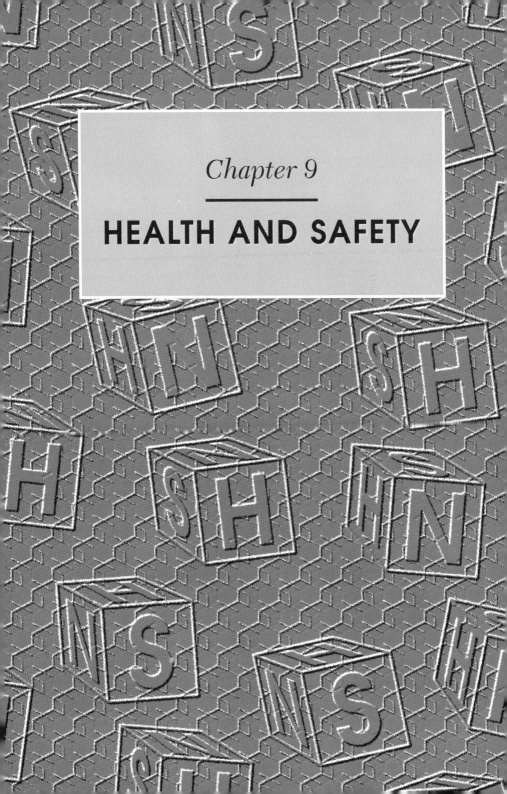

# Chapter 9

## HEALTH AND SAFETY

## THE HEALTH AND SAFETY COMMISSION

The main body to give guidance on health and safety is the Health and Safety Commission. In turn, it takes advice from its own agency, the Health Services Advisory Committee. Membership of the committee is nominated by NHS management, professional associations, trade unions and the private sector.

The Commission's operational arm, the Health and Safety Executive (HSE) has a health review group which is responsible for providing advice to HSE inspectors who visit health-care establishments. The HSE also provides a great deal of information on occupational health and safety. The main statute concerned with occupational health and safety is the *Health and Safety at Work Act* 1974 (HSWA).

Inspection of buildings under the HSWA is carried out by inspectors of the HSE, except in the case of separately sited office and residential accommodation where inspections are carried out by local authorities. However, the HSWA does not cover food hygiene or general matters relating to fires.

The HSWA details general guidelines for both employers and employees. Over the years, a number of regulations have been made under the Act including:

- dealing with safety representatives and safety committees
- reporting of injuries
- diseases and dangerous occurrences
- first-aid
- hazardous and dangerous substances.

The Act applies to almost every employer and employee, and to most NHS premises.

## OCCUPATIONAL HEALTH

The main objectives of the occupational health service are:

- To promote and maintain the highest possible level of health, both physical and mental, for all employees, and to determine whether they are physically and mentally fit for the job in which they are engaged.
- To safeguard staff from hazards arising from their work or from the environment in which they operate, by means of accident prevention, environment control and the prevention of serious illness. Also to provide emergency treatment to staff becoming ill at work, and to give assistance with their subsequent rehabilitation after illness or surgery.

In the past, it can be said that the occupational health department (OHD) mainly concentrated on the more physical aspects of employment. In the future it is hoped, however, that greater emphasis will be placed on more preventive areas, such as health assessments and health screening.

As many employees could be suspicious that a referral to the OHD might result in the end of their employment, it is essential that these departments are seen as being entirely independent and professional in their work.

In an ideal situation, therefore, the building in which the OHD is situated should offer those visiting it a confidential atmosphere for private clinical examinations.

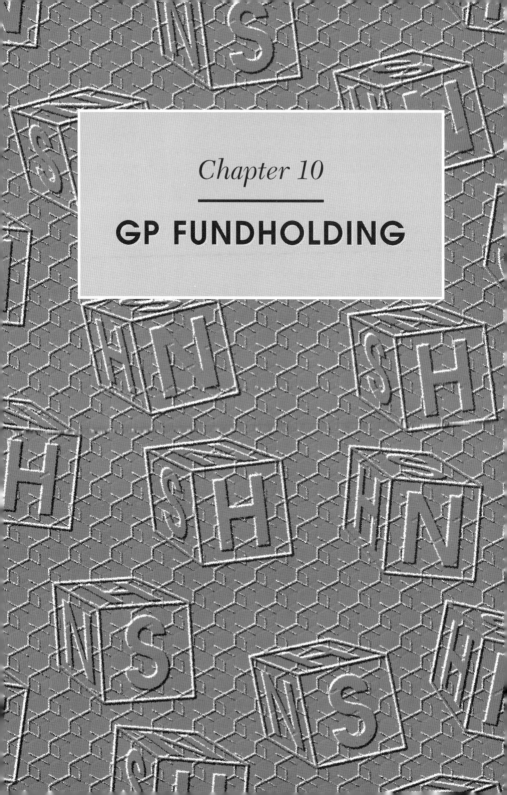

# Chapter 10

## GP FUNDHOLDING

## THE SCHEME IN GENERAL

The GP fundholding scheme allows general practitioners direct control of budgets for the purchase of drugs, staff, and hospital and community services to meet the health needs of their practice population.

It is widely believed that the fundholding scheme has considerably influenced the delivery and quality of hospital and community health services for the patients of fundholding and non-fundholding GPs alike, for example by the reduction in waiting-list times.

Allowing GPs control over their own budgets also enables innovative developments to take place within general practice for the benefit and convenience of patients, such as the provision of paramedical services and outpatient facilities located within GP surgeries.

### What a fundholding budget covers

GP fundholding budgets cover three main areas of expenditure:

  a) A defined range of hospital and community health services.
  b) Prescribing costs.
  c) Practice staff.

Fundholders may move (subject to HA approval) monies from one budget to another as they judge most appropriate to meet patient needs.

## WHAT SERVICES CAN GP FUNDHOLDERS PURCHASE?

Hospital and community health services:

- Inpatients - defined elective inpatient and day-case treatment.
- Outpatients - majority of outpatient attendances.
- Community health services.
- Domiciliary consultations.
- Direct-access therapy services.
- Direct-access tests and investigations - diagnostic tests and investigations except breast screening by mammography and cervical cytology carried out under the call and recall scheme.

### Prescribing

Fundholders are also set budgets for the cost of drugs prescribed for their patients. These are largely based on historical prescribing patterns using the capitation data (the number and age of patients on a GP list). The same basis is used when calculating budgets for non-fundholding practices. Arrangements for setting budgets may well vary from year to year.

### Practice staff

A proportion (70% of salaries and 100% of National Insurance contributions) of the cost of staff directly employed by the practice is reimbursed by the HA. This process of reimbursement is also the same for non-fundholding practices. Some HAs may have calculated this on a capitation basis with each patient on a GP's list being worth a specified amount of money.

In return, fundholders are required to:

- Produce development plans outlining the practice's purchasing intentions.
- Provide certain information returns, usually computer-generated.
- Monitor provider (usually Trust) performance against contracts.
- Manage expenditure against budgets.
- Operate the fundholding computer system.
- Work co-operatively with local Health Authority purchasers.

## FUNDHOLDING CRITERIA

Purchasers who wish to become fundholders are required to satisfy the following statutory requirements:

a) Practices must have a list size (separately or combined with other practices) of at least 5,000 patients for standard fundholding and 3,000 patients for community fundholding.

b) Practices must be, or be taking steps to become, computerised.

c) Practices must demonstrate a capability, or potential, to manage large sums of money.

### How the budget is calculated

Hospital and community health services are calculated on the basis of activity data recorded by practices in their preparatory year. The preparatory year is the year immediately preceding the first year of fundholding. Future budgets may be adjusted in the light of inflation and significant changes in list size, or if significant errors in the original activity data are detected.

### Other allowances

In recognition of the additional demands placed upon GP fundholders, allowances for management time and computing costs are available under the scheme. At the time of writing, a maximum allowance of £21,255 is available in the preparatory year plus £650 if they have a branch surgery. There is also a computing allowance to cover 100% reimbursement of software and 75% reimbursement of hardware for the installation of a computerised accounting system to monitor referrals and expenditure. In subsequent years they may bid for additional equipment from the Health Authority which is subject to available funds.

Following the preparatory year, a management allowance, usually staff-oriented to cover the cost of managing the fundholding budget, of up to £27,258 plus a variable amount dependent on list size, is payable to fundholding practices. Fundholders must meet the on-going maintenance costs of their fundholding systems from their management allowance.

## What is excluded from the fundholding scheme?

The hospital services element of the scheme is limited to certain inpatient and day-case treatment. The following services are specifically excluded from the scheme:

- accident and emergency
- maternity services
- chemotherapy treatment
- radiotherapy treatment
- renal dialysis
- self-referrals to hospital.

## Areas in which fundholding practices may use savings from their budgets

At the end of the financial year, fundholding accounts are subject to audit by the Audit Commission. Once audited, any savings may be used by the practice in compliance with current fundholding regulations for the benefit of patients. The savings could be used for the purchase of:

- additional staff or staff time
- additional hospital and community health services
- additional prescribing
- improvements to practice premises
- improvements to patient facilities
- the provision of additional medical equipment
- paramedical services on site.

In conclusion, GP fundholders can be compared with HAs, as both are purchasers negotiating contracts with the provider units for the provision of health care for their population.

## EFFECTS OF THE SCHEME

In the first year of the scheme, 7% of the population were cared for by fundholding GPs. In the second year this figure had risen to 14%, and by the time the sixth wave of fundholders had joined the scheme it had reached 50%.

The spread of fundholding is extremely varied, with some areas being almost completely fundholding, while in others it is less prevalent.

## COMMUNITY FUNDHOLDING

Practices with a list size of 3,000 patients or above can apply to join the community fundholding scheme. This scheme excludes all elective surgery and outpatient appointments that are included in the current form of fundholding. It does, however, give practices the opportunity to hold their own budgets for prescribing, staff, community health services and diagnostic tests (see Box 8).

Community fundholders are expected to negotiate contracts with local providers for the provision of community health services and diagnostic tests. In line with standard fundholders, community fundholders will probably elect to hold block contracts for these services due to the quantity of work involved in monitoring diagnostic tests and the current lack of information surrounding community nursing work. The community fundholding drugs budget is set in exactly the same way as for other non-fundholding GPs under the indicative prescribing scheme. Expenditure in the previous year is used as the base figure, then adjusted by reference to the responsible Authority's average prescribing costs, high cost patients and ASTRO-PUs.

Staff costs are reimbursed in the same way as for non-fundholding GPs, i.e. 70% of salary and 100% employer's N.I. costs. A management allowance is also available to cover the cost of additional staff taken on to facilitate the fundholding process.

The funding for the diagnostic tests in the community fundholding budget is deducted from the Health Authority's allocation and re-allocated to the GP fundholding practice. The Authority acts as a paymaster for the practice and pays the bills from the provider units. The Health Authority also pays the drugs bill on behalf of the fundholders, the staffing element and management allowance.

---

## BOX 8  THE ELEMENTS OF THE COMMUNITY FUNDHOLDING SCHEME

The budget is composed of three elements:

- diagnostic tests, direct-access services and community care;
- prescribing budget;
- staff costs.

In-hospital services:

- diagnostic tests;
- direct-access services including physiotherapy, chiropody, speech therapy and dietetics
- community care including district nurses, health visitors.

---

## TOTAL PURCHASING

At the time of publication this scheme was being piloted. Total purchasing allows GPs to purchase all hospital and community health services for their patients.

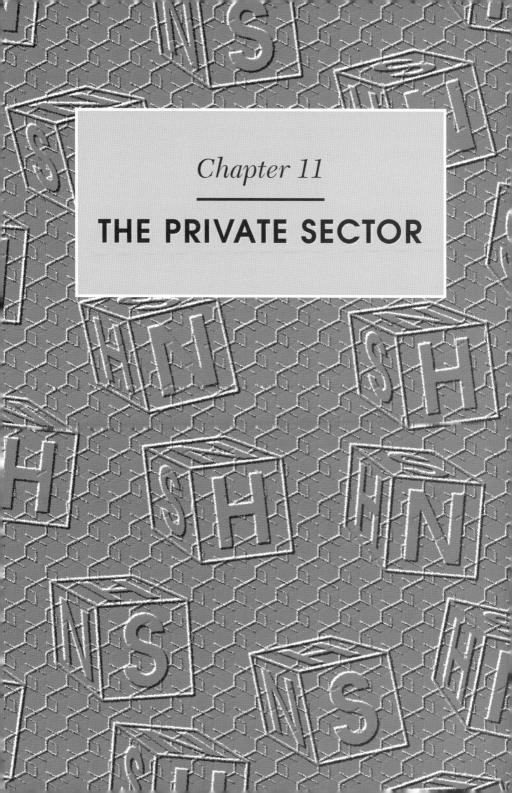

*Chapter 11*

# THE PRIVATE SECTOR

It is difficult to compare the independent sector with the NHS; however, on a financial basis, a direct comparison between combined acute and non-acute hospital and nursing home care reveals the following net revenue and capital costs for combined acute and non-acute hospital and nursing home care for 1994:

£ 5,000,000          The independent sector
£21,500,000         NHS hospital services

Although a few charitable or non-affiliated hospitals remain, most independent hospitals now belong to one of the three major groups: the BMI (British Medical International) group, British United Provident Association (BUPA) and Nuffield.

It is interesting to note that many insurers are now operating in a very similar manner to NHS purchasers, in attempting to pre-authorise claims prior to submission, and monitor treatment to ensure it conforms to an agreed protocol.

One area of the private sector which appears to be increasing is the psychiatric sector. This area has grown rapidly because of the reduction in the number of large NHS psychiatric hospitals. It is fair to say, however, that with regard to acute hospital services, purchasers of NHS care still contract in the main with NHS providers and not the independent sector, although occasionally some Health Authorities will contract care of their elderly patients to independent nursing homes.

In recent years, the independent sector has started to face some opposition, especially from NHS Trusts who have opened an increasing number of dedicated units which will only treat private patients.

## CONSULTANTS IN PRIVATE PRACTICE

Full-time NHS consultants are allowed to practise privately and earn up to 10% in addition to their NHS salary. In reality, this can be extremely difficult to monitor.

There is, however, no restriction on the amount of private practice undertaken by part-time NHS consultants. Most consultants in private practice have a number of 'rooms' from which they practise. In addition, many will employ a secretary and/or receptionist.

Private consultations are usually arranged by appointment, and most appointments are made by the patient's GP, but sometimes are arranged by the patients themselves. If, after the first consultation, hospital treatment is needed, the patient may elect to have this either privately or via the NHS.

Many consultants working in private practice specialise in one of the following disciplines:

- Cardiology - disorders of the human heart.
- Dermatology - diseases of the skin.

- Obstetrics and gynaecology - this largely involves care of the expectant mother and diseases of the female reproductive system.
- Neurology - disorders of the nervous system which have been caused by injury or disease.
- Ophthalmology - function and disorders of the eye.
- Otorhinolaryngology - examination and treatment of the ear, nose and throat.
- Paediatrics - diseases and disorders in children.
- Geriatric medicine - special diseases and problems which are associated with elderly patients.
- Psychiatry - this specialty is wide-ranging and will cover mental health problems in all age groups.

Other specialties include orthopaedics, plastic surgery, gastroenterology and so on.

## 'COMPLEMENTARY' TREATMENT

In addition to the more conventional forms of private medicine, there has been a sharp increase in the promotion and use of complementary (previously referred to as 'alternative') therapies. In many instances, these combine with more conventional NHS treatments.

A brief guide to the more high profile services which are currently available is given here.

### Acupuncture

Medical acupuncture involves the release of natural pain killers (endorphins) by needles activating deep sensory nerves. Acupuncture is often used to treat migraine, arthritis, back pain, sports injuries, anxiety, depression, hayfever and eczema.

In some instances, acupuncture is used in smoking cessation and weight loss. Acupuncture is not, however, used for acute surgical conditions. Many GPs include acupuncture in day-to-day NHS practice in addition to the services offered by private acupuncturists.

The British Medical Acupuncture Society (BMAS) gives basic training to doctors and also provides intermediate and advanced courses (see Useful Addresses).

### Alexander Technique

The Alexander Technique is a method of psychophysical re-education which has therapeutic benefits. It encourages individuals to take responsibility for their own health and well-being by becoming aware of how they are using themselves in their everyday activities.

Alexander Technique teachers will point out the patterns of tension and collapse which interfere with the body's natural balance and co-ordination. These patterns put unrestricted strain and pressures on the body, and are thought to lead to a decrease in general functioning with time. Alexander Techniques can be used to alleviate the problems of stress and pain, especially musculoskeletal pain, such as neck and back problems.

All teachers have undertaken a three-year full-time course of training, which is monitored by the Society of Teachers of the Alexander Technique (STAT).

Interestingly, some GP fundholders have employed Alexander teachers. Non-fundholders can, if they so wish, apply to the HA in line with other complementary therapies. In addition, BUPA, and other insurance companies, may pay for a course of lessons if a patient is referred by a GP or consultant.

## Aromatherapy

Aromatherapy involves the use of aromatic substances, usually oils, applied through various methods including massage, baths, compresses and inhalation.

The oils are used to aid pain relief, help with relaxation and encourage a sense of calm and well-being. Aromatherapy is deemed to be particularly effective in the treatment of stress-related conditions, such as panic attacks, headaches, insomnia and hypertension. It is also thought to help those who suffer from arthritis and rheumatism.

Qualified aromatherapists have been trained in the chemistry, properties, uses and application of essential oils. They will also have undertaken training in massage.

Aromatherapy is usually available through private practice and natural-health centres. However, because of recently increased demand, some aromatherapists have started to work in day centres, hospitals, hospices and even some GP practices.

## Chiropractic

Chiropractic is a manipulative therapy. Treatment often involves making adjustments to stiff or irritated joints. The more common complaints which can be treated by chiropractors are low back pain, sciatic pain, neck, shoulder or arm pain, and sports injuries.

Members of the British Chiropractic Association have completed a full-time five-year degree course. Graduating students are required to undertake a further one-year postgraduate programme at a regional centre.

A few fundholding practices have purchased the service of chiropractors. However, HA permission has first to be granted. It is possible at a later date that chiropractic treatment may be provided for fundholders via the British Chiropractic Association.

## Herbal medicine

It is interesting to note that a quarter of modern orthodox drugs are still derived from plant medicine.

The patients who are referred to herbal practitioners are often those suffering from migraine, arthritis and skin disorders.

Members of the National Institute of Medical Herbalists have undertaken a four-year training period. In addition, herbal practitioners are trained to recognise acute and chronic diseases and refer them to a GP. Most practitioners work in the private sector; however, there are a few who offer NHS treatment.

## Homeopathy

The essential basis of homeopathy is that the medicines are similar to the symptoms they are used to treat, an example being the use of amphetamines to treat hyperactive children.

Training in this kind of therapy varies, although a GP can be qualified through the Faculty of Homeopathy.

Homeopathy is practised in primary care, where it provides an alternative to the treatment of such conditions as coughs and sore throats. Chronic or recurrent disorders, such as asthma, migraine and arthritis, can also be treated.

Some homeopathic medicines can be prescribed on the NHS, and some GPs use homeopathy. In addition, many medical homeopaths work exclusively in private practice. There are currently five homeopathic hospitals in London, Glasgow, Liverpool, Bristol and Tunbridge Wells.

## Reflexology

Reflexology is the art of applying manual pressure to the feet. It is based on the idea that specific foot reflexes correspond to various organs and structures of the body. Reflexology is often used to treat 'stress-related conditions' and musculoskeletal problems, and has also been found useful in obstetrics. Reflexologists will have completed a course of instruction, which includes practical work and home study. At the moment, it is extremely unusual for reflexology to be available under the NHS.

## Shiatsu

Shiatsu works on the body's natural energy network. It involves the use of fingers, thumbs and palms in conjunction with general stretching. Although Shiatsu involves working on the body with the hands, patients undergoing Shiatsu treatment remain fully clothed. Shiatsu can relieve many problems such as nausea, vomiting and diarrhoea. It is also deemed to be effective in the treatment of headaches, colds and flus etc.

Entry to the Shiatsu Society Register means that a practitioner must have completed 500 hours of training, and studied for a minimum of three years at a recognised school with a recognised Shiatsu teacher.

Most registered practitioners do not provide NHS services.

# USEFUL ADDRESSES

Alcoholics Anonymous (General Service Board) PO Box 1 Stonebow House Stonebow YORK YO1 2NJ Tel: 01904 644 026

British Medical Acupuncture Society (BMAS) Newton House Newton Lane Whitley WARRINGTON WA4 4JA Tel: 01925 737 0727

British Medical Association (BMA) BMA House Tavistock Square LONDON WC1H 9JP Tel: 0171 387 4499

Cancer Relief Macmillan Fund 15/19 Britten Street LONDON SW3 3TY Tel: 0171 351 7811

Chiropractic Advancement Association 56 Barnes Crescent WIMBOURNE Dorset BH21 2AZ

Department of Health Richmond House 79 Whitehall LONDON WC1H 9TX

Health Education Authority Hamilton House Mabledon Place LONDON WC1H 9TX Tel: 0171 383 3833

MIND (National Association for Mental Health) 22 Harley Street LONDON W1N 2ED

National Association of Fundholding Practices 12 Durham Road Raynes Park LONDON SW20 0TD Tel: 0181 944 7945

National Blood Transfusion Centre Gateway House Picadilly South MANCHESTER M60 7LP Tel: 0161 273 7181

National Institute of Medical Herbalists 56 Longbrook Street EXETER Devon EX4 6AH Tel: 01392 426 022

RNIB (Royal National Institute for the Blind) 224 Great Portland Street LONDON W1N 6AA Tel: 0171 388 1266

RNID (Royal National Institute for the Deaf) 105 Gower Street LONDON WC1E 6AH Tel: 0171 383 3154

Terence Higgins Trust 52-54 Gray's Inn Rd LONDON WC1X 8JU Tel: 0171 242 1010

United Kingdom Central Council for Nursing, Midwifery and Health Visiting 23 Portland Place LONDON W1N 3AF

# BIBLIOGRAPHY

Department of Health. *The Patients' Charter.* London: DoH, 1991 (EL(91)128).

Department of Health. *The Children Act.* London: HMSO, 1989.

Department of Health. *The Children Act 1989 - an introductory guide for the NHS.* London: Health Publications Unit, 1991.

Department of Health. *Changing childbirth.* London: HMSO, 1993.

Department of Health. *Mental Health Act for England and Wales.* London: HMSO, 1983.

Great Britain Parliament. *National Health Service and Community Care Act.* London: HMSO, 1990.

Department of Health. *Caring for people: community care in the next decade and beyond.* London: HMSO, 1989.

Department of Health. *Working for patients.* London: HMSO, 1989.

Health Departments of Great Britain. *General Practice in the National Health Service. The 1990 Contract.* London: HMSO, 1989.

Health and Safety Commission. *Health and Safety at Work Act.* London: HMSO, 1974.

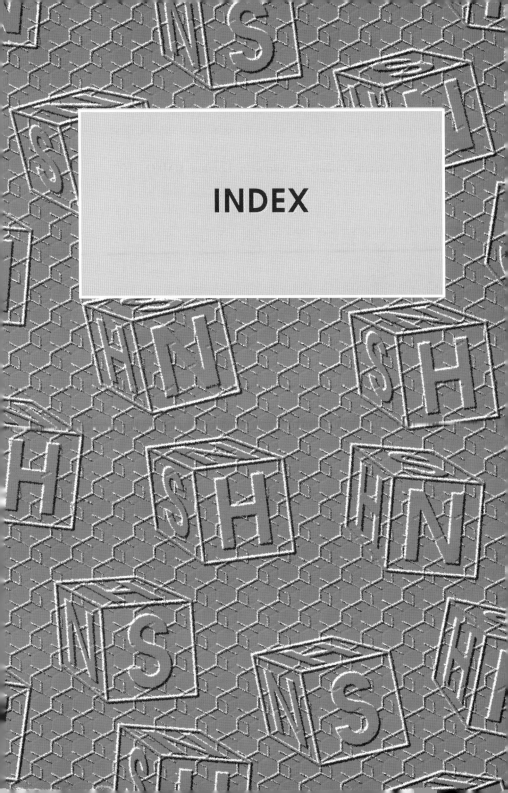

# INDEX

## A

Accident & emergency departments
32, 33, 44, 46, 54, 86
Acupuncture - British Medical
Society 91
Adoption 66
AIDS 22, 66, 69, 70
Alexander Technique - Society of
Teachers of 91, 92
Alcohol abuse 66
Alcoholics Anonymous 69
Aled Richards Trust 69
Ambulance Services 10, 54
emergency & urgent 55
Antenatal care 59
Aromatherapy 92
Audit Commission 24, 86

## B

Bereavement counsellor 74
Breast-care adviser 73
Breast screening 38, 84
Blood transfusion services 55, 56, 58

## C

Cancer Relief MacMillan Fund 74
Cancer Relief MacMillan Nurses 74
Capital charges 22
Capitation 38, 39, 84, 85
Cervical cytology 36, 38, 58, 84
Chaplains 74
Changing Childbirth 60
Charge nurse 62
Chief Executives
HA 30
NHSE 14, 17, 20
Trusts 42
Chief Medical Officer (NHSE) 14
Child health services 56-58

clinics 57
computer system 39, 69
immunisation 39, 56
preschool 39
surveillance 39, 56, 57
Surveillance Register 57
Children Act 1989 57-58, 67
Children (Secure Accomodation)
Regulations 58
Chiropractic - British Association of 92
Chiropodists 50
Clinical chemistry 58
Clearing house system 27
Clinical directorates (Trusts) 42, 44
Clinical directors 42
Clinical liaison groups 42, 51
Clinical waste 40
Community care 70
Community Care Act 1990 67
Community fundholding 84, 86-87
Community Health Councils (CHCs)
26, 31, 36, 51, 75, 76
Community health services 42, 43,
84-87
Community and Mental Health
Directorate 42
Community needle & exchange
scheme 35
Community nursing contracts 63
Community nursing sister, See district
nurse
Community paediatricians 56, 69
Community psychiatric nurses 60, 73
Complaints 30, 31, 34, 36, 61, 76
Complementary treatment 91-93
Computerised tomography 46
Consultants 90, 91
Contracting Directorate (HAs) 31,
32-34, 37
Communicable diseases 40
Consumer services departments
(HAs) 36
Contracts 22, 31-35, 38-40

## N

National Association of Health
Authorities & Trusts (NAHAT) 51
National Blood Authority (NBA) 14,
28, 55
National Council for Voluntary
Organisations 77
National Vocational Qualification
(NVQ) 54
NHS
Chief Executive 14, 17, 20
Executive 14-17, 26-28
Policy Board 17
Regional Directors 17, 26
Supplies Authority 14
Training Directorate 54
Trusts 10, 14, 17, 18, 20, 22, 24, 26,
27, 32-35, 41-52, 54, 57, 68,
90
Wales and Scotland 19, 20
Night visit fees 39
Non-executive directors 17
Nurse practitioners 62
Nurse prescribing 63
Nursing homes
Registration and inspection of 33, 34
*Registration of Nursing Homes Act
1984* 34
Nursing services 60-63

## O

Obstetricians 59
Ombudsman 24
Open health 27
Operating theatres 47
Opticians 36, 75
Outbreak control plans 40
Occupational health 80, 81
Occupational therapists 48
Outpatient departments 44, 46, 49
Out-of-hours services 67

## P

Paediatric nurse 73
Paediatricians 56
Paramedics 55
Patients
*Charter* 11, 27, 33, 54, 56, 98
registration of 38
representative 51
Permanent secretary 14
Personnel & training department
(HAs) 36
Pharmaceutical Adviser (HAs) 36
Pharmacists 38, 39, 75
Physiotherapists 48, 49
Play groups 68
Policy Board 14
Postgraduate Education Allowance
39
Postnatal care 59, 60
Practice
annual reports 35
managers 72
nurses 72
nurse trainers 74
staff budgets 84
staff/premises adviser 38
Preschool child health 39
Prescribing 84
Primary Health & Community Group
(CHC) 75
Primary health-care services 70-74
Primary health-care teams 48, 50, 61,
70-74
Primary health-care nursing 62, 70-74
Primary nursing 63
Private sector 88-93
Probation officers 70
Project 2000 63
Providers 17, 27, 67, 68, 86, 90
Public Accounts Committee 24
Public Expenditure Survey (PES) 22